On the Palm of His Hand

Within the pages of [this little book] one will find that Marion Levandowski has shared the moving memory of a very special friend's journey of faith, suffering and love. It is a vivid portrait of a personality—Phyllis—who touched many lives and knew well the taste of both laughter and sorrow.　　　Rev. Michael Mannion, S.T.L., M.A.

Founder and Director, Discovery Retreat Program

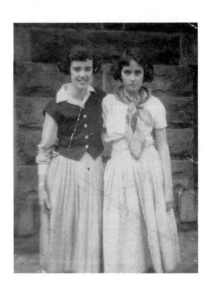

(Top) Marion (*left*) and Phyllis in 8th grade, 1950, and (below) 25 years later: Phyllis (*left*) and Marion.

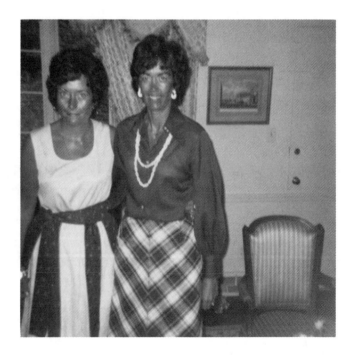

On the Palm of His Hand

Marion Lee Levandowski

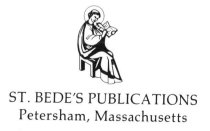

ST. BEDE'S PUBLICATIONS
Petersham, Massachusetts

Cover design by Celine McManamon and Bernadette Jaeger, OSB

LIBRARY OF CONGRESS CATALOGING-IN-PUBLICATION DATA

Levandowski, Marion Lee, 1936-
  On the palm of His hand.

  1. Fleck, Phyllis—Health. 2. Cancer—Patients—United
States—Biography. 3. Cancer—Religious aspects—Catholic
Church. I. Title.
RC265.6.F57L48   1987   282'.092'4   [B]   87-32361
ISBN 0-932506-62-3

Published by   St. Bede's Publications
               P.O. Box 545
               Petersham, Massachusetts 01366-0545

Contents

Acknowledgments

A special thank you to Larry Weber, whose unselfish concern for my friend Phyllis prompted him to suggest I invite her to New Jersey. That suggestion materialized into her visit, and that visit poured a shower of blessings on many people. Hopefully, more lives will be touched by this story, creating a continuous flow of blessings.

I would also like to express my sincere appreciation to Rev. Edward D. O'Connor, CSC, Professor of Theology, Notre Dame University, and Sr. Mary Schmidt, past President and Professor of English, Seton Hill College. Each of them was kind enough to read my manuscript, and their encouragement and suggestions were extremely helpful.

While this story is about an old and cherished friend, I am deeply indebted to a new and cherished friend, Elvira Brown. Not only did she play a prominent role in the story, her contribution to every phase of this endeavor turned a dream into a reality. This effort is my "maiden voyage" and the experience of putting the book together is a story in itself. Elvira also has the dubious distinction of introducing me to the wondrous world of computers—the twentieth century marvel that makes the mechanics of writing a pleasure.

To you alone, O Lord,
    to you alone,
and not to us, must glory
    be given
because of your constant love
    and faithfulness.
Psalm 115:1

The Mourning

Those whom the Lord has ransomed will
return, crowned with everlasting joy;
sorrow and mourning will flee.
Isaiah 35:10

It was one of the saddest days of my life. As I looked at the faces of my friends around me, I couldn't help thinking about how many times, as children, we had knelt together side by side. Only *this* day was different—this day we were mourning the loss of Phyllis, a beloved lifelong friend. The bond of friendship she and I had shared was unique—it had survived forty years, despite the fact that we had been geographically separated for more than twenty-five of those years. Now there was a void in that bond and it would never be the same.

The priest stood at the foot of the altar waiting for the procession and the casket carrying her body. I pondered on how ritual is part and parcel of our life in the Church. From beginning to end, our lives are measured in these sacramental rites.

I had known Phyllis from the time we made our First Holy Communion together. How tender and innocent we were then. We giggled our way through grade school, and during those painful adolescent years we shared what we thought at the time were earth-shattering secrets. After school days, a time when many friends drift apart, we became even closer, sharing our hopes and dreams for the future.

Phyllis's dream came true the day she became engaged to

a young man named Chuck. From their first meeting she knew he was the one. There were many eligible men vying for her attention, but I can still hear her telling me how she prayed nightly that Chuck would be the man with whom she would share her life. It was not until two years later, though, that a serious commitment developed, and in a matter of months they wed.

At the time of her marriage, I was working in Washington, D.C., but returned home to take part in this joyous occasion in her life. The ceremony, another milestone marked by ritual, was spectacular. Except for the long-stemmed red roses the bridesmaids carried, it was an all white wedding, and she was an exquisitely beautiful bride.

I now watched in disbelief while the priest sprinkled her coffin with holy water. "In the name of the Father and of the Son and of the Holy Spirit..."

*　　　*　　　*

It was an afternoon in May when the news first reached me—the news that Phyllis had cancer. I had just returned from the supermarket. Juggling groceries while scrambling for the door key, my daughter rushed to the rescue.

"Mom, your friend Nancy from Pittsburgh called—wants you to call her back. Says it's very important!"

When Nancy finished telling me how Phyllis had discovered a lump, that it was malignant, and that she was slated for surgery, my immediate reaction was, "I can't believe this has happened—she is too beautiful," as if her beauty could repel such an ugly disease. I knew I had to pull myself together and call her, but what does one say to a dear friend in such a dreadful situation? My anxiety was in vain because when I finally called her, she was in remarkably good spirits.

I remember saying, "Phyllis, you're very fortunate because you have always had such a strong faith—all you have to do now is tap into that faith."

"I know," she agreed. "I've already asked my surgeon to wear a relic of St. John Neumann." She explained that miraculous cures, often of cancer, were attributed to the intercession of this saint.

While the surgery was indeed successful, she still had to endure the discomfort of chemotherapy which would be followed by radiation. She went to California to recuperate, and I began to pray that the surgery and subsequent therapy would totally erase any trace of the disease.

*   *   *

Here we were, two years later, at her funeral, each of us in our own way nurturing memories of this beautiful friend who was gone. As for me, I was struck by the stark contrast between the seriousness of the funeral service and the wit and warmth of Phyllis. At the sound of the somber words from the priest, my mind wandered back to another occasion when we were kneeling together in church.

We were kids at the time, always ready for a new adventure, and decided one Saturday night that it might be fun to go into the heart of the city to a 2:00 A.M. Mass. Since none of us was properly dressed for Mass (in those days, slacks were not acceptable attire and a hat was absolutely essential), we raided the closet of our hostess. Imagine six girls ranging from 5'1" to 5'9" wearing the same size? It made for some pretty interesting outfits!

This particular Mass attracted a wide variety of the faithful: night shift people, show biz types, policemen, firemen, cabbies, and assorted derelicts. It was quite an array and in our ill-fitting clothes we blended in beautifully. I was busy gawking at the odd assortment of people entering the church when Phyllis poked my elbow. There, in the pew in front of us, were several men in various stages of inebriation: one sleeping, another hanging onto the railing, one resting his head on the shoulder of another. She rolled her eyes, pursed her lips, and, with a very officious nod, whispered, "I see the Holy Name Society is represented!" It was vintage Phyllis—she never missed an opportunity to poke fun at the ridiculous.

But there was no humor, no warmth here today, save for memories. For me, one of the great blessings of the Roman Catholic Faith lies in the liturgy of the Mass. The mystery that takes place on the altar is in no way affected by the personality or style of the priest. However, on this day, I selfishly longed for a golden-tongued orator who would capture the essence of my beloved friend. Instead, I heard the droning voice of a priest who sounded so harsh, so doleful—so unlike Phyllis. I was hoping for words of comfort, but he was scolding us, lecturing us.

I began to squirm in my seat, shaking my head and wondering "Why?" I realized if she were sitting next to me, she would have poked fun at the irony of the situation. Then I heard him bellow, "You must all *pray* for the soul of Phyllis...."

When was it, I thought to myself, that I first began to pray seriously for Phyllis? Looking back, I believe it happened the summer following her surgery. I was traveling with my family in Canada and we were so charmed by Quebec that we stayed on an extra day. The famous Shrine of St. Anne de Beaupré was just outside of Quebec, and I asked my husband, Ed, to take me there. Never having seen a shrine, I thought it would be an interesting experience for the whole family and it would give me the opportunity to offer a special prayer for Phyllis. I had no knowledge of the Shrine, other than that it was noted for miraculous cures. This merely served to pique my curiosity.

Even though the Shrine is in a nondescript little village, it is located right off a major highway; the lot was already filled with cars and buses when we arrived. We couldn't help but be impressed by the massive size of the basilica itself and the grounds surrounding the church which were perfectly landscaped with tall, stately trees, brightly-colored flowers, and lush manicured lawns. On one side of the parking lot, before we reached the Shrine, we saw the hospital where the physical and spiritual needs of the sick are met. We learned that patients there are cared for by the finest doctors and also prayed over for healing.

We noticed a crowd gathered outside in front of the church. Drawing closer, we realized it was a procession of pilgrims making the Stations of the Cross, following the path up a steep hill where life-size bronze statues depicting the passion and death of our Lord dotted the hillside. The people were led by a priest who intoned prayers in French at the foot of each station.

After climbing the dozens of gray stone steps leading to the church, the first things we noticed upon entering were two enormous columns covered from floor to ceiling with crutches, braces, pictures, and so on—all documenting miraculous cures brought about through the intercession of St. Anne.

In hushed tones I told Ed that I wanted to light a candle for Phyllis. Slowly, I walked down the center aisle, scanning the breathtakingly beautiful marble altars with their finely chiseled statues on both sides of the basilica. The main nave was supported with splendidly carved pillars and columns. Above the columns and surrounding the basilica, my eyes feasted on the magnificent array of stained glass windows, each affording a visual portrayal of Holy Scripture. Then my eyes fell upon a fountain, situated near the main altar. Its white marble glistened in the glow of candlelight. Rising up in the center of the fountain, atop an onyx pedestal, was an eight-foot statue of St. Anne with the child Mary resting on her right arm. Both were crowned with jewels.

I was amused at my own ignorance—somehow it had never occurred to me that St. Anne de Beaupré was *the* St. Anne, mother of Mary and grandmother of Jesus.

I lit a candle and knelt down at the railing which surrounded the fountain. Watching the flickering flame create a warm glow, I could actually feel the burning desire inside me for God to heal Phyllis.

I picked up the prayer card in front of me, and suddenly I remembered something I had all but forgotten. Nineteen years earlier, this very prayer was the one I had recited while making a novena. It was a powerful prayer and the answer had been swift. I had been faced with a serious problem at the time, one I felt ill-equipped to solve objectively. Not knowing whom to turn to, I confided in Phyllis and she recommended St. Anne to me. Giving me a prayer card bearing a picture of this same statue, she said, "Marion, recite this prayer in faith and humility, and I promise you St. Anne will intercede for you." I eagerly snatched the card from her hand as I promised to follow her advice, and each morning for nine days I went to Mass and Holy Communion, fervently asking St. Anne to grant my request.

Now, gazing down at the laminated card in front of me, not only did I recall the speed with which my prayer had been answered, but also the benefits that were evident even to this day! And it was Phyllis who had coaxed me to stick with prayer—who imparted to me the confidence to believe in the power of prayer. Remembering it now, after all these years, was no small thing. I felt that our prayer had come full circle. It was apparent to me that this was not a coincidence, but that God was beginning to teach me the importance of intercessory prayer.

It was a moment that had to be shared, and when I later told Phyllis how clearly this all came back to me while kneeling at the fountain in prayer for her, she was thrilled. Not only that—she had a surprise for me. While I was away, St. Anne was present in her thoughts too, first by a prayer card which was sent to her through the mail, and then by another, more personal incident.

"You're not going to believe this, Marion, but a few weeks ago, my father-in-law made a special pilgrimage to that very shrine to pray for my recovery!"

It was after this experience that I began to pray in earnest for her—and I also prevailed upon the people in my prayer group to pray as well.

Phyllis began radiation treatment and continued to keep in touch by phone frequently. After Christmas, she came to New Jersey for a few days and stayed with her sister Ann. The primary purpose of her trip was to consult another doctor—she and Chuck wanted to avail themselves of everything new in the field. This gave me an opportunity to visit with her since I lived only twenty minutes away.

When I saw her, I was startled by her appearance. She was still as lovely as ever. There was no hint in her countenance of what she had been through. Her almost black hair was swept away from her face, emphasizing her classic features—high cheekbones, long thin nose, and delicate mouth. Her eyes, her most outstanding feature, were clear and bright, with their brilliant shade of blue accented by her long, full eyelashes.

The consultation with the doctor created a great deal of anxiety since he did not agree with the therapy she was receiving. After returning home, she became frightened, uncertain how to proceed. While I understood her desire to explore other avenues, the risk that she might lose confidence in her primary doctors was a concern to me.

* * *

That seemed such a short time ago, and here I was kneeling at her funeral, heartbroken and confused, trying to piece together all the events leading up to this moment.

The Mass was drawing to a close. The pallbearers left their pews once again and placed themselves into position at the foot of the altar. They slowly passed in front of us bearing the coffin. Her husband, children, and family followed in mournful silence. Then quietly and reverently, the rest of us left the church and lined up in our cars for the long drive to the cemetery. There was to be no graveside ceremony; instead we congregated in a small chapel for our last goodbye. We formed a semicircle behind the priest, who read aloud the prayers for the faithful departed, once again sprinkling holy water.

It was over—just like that. I glanced over at Chuck who broke into sobs as he placed his hand tenderly on the casket one last time. His father embraced him and, arm in arm, they walked to the waiting limousine.

It was more than I could bear. I turned and walked away from the circle of friends, filled with such sorrow, such anguish. My life had been so intertwined with Phyllis, with her illness, with the ever-constant hope that she would recover, she would live. Now it was over. What did it all mean?

It was this illness that had actively brought me back into her life. So much had happened during that time; I knew I would never be the same. Looking back now, I count it a rare privilege that I was allowed to play a role in her "agony in the garden." It was an intensely personal experience, but as a tribute to my precious friend, I would like to share that special time with others. This, then, is a story of friendship, of hope, of acceptance, and of thanksgiving, but most of all, this is a story of God's perfect love.

The Search

I sought the Lord and He answered me
and delivered me from all my fears.
Psalm 34:5

In the early spring of 1984 Phyllis called, and the moment I heard her voice I knew something had changed. She broke into sobs as she told me the awful news—the cancer had returned! She had opted for a lumpectomy on the first surgery and now, one year later, a tumor was found in the same area. A mastectomy was no longer a matter of choice. Hearing the despair in her voice, I tried to offer comfort and strength with the reminder of how much God loved her. Having experienced two miracles in my own life (events which Phyllis was aware of), I assured her that miracles really do happen and together we would ask God to touch her with His healing power.

This latest setback shattered what little confidence she still had in her doctors, and so she put herself into the care of a new team. At the same time, Chuck was more determined than ever to investigate every available therapy. He wanted to leave no stone unturned in his effort to do everything humanly possible to save Phyllis. He even paid his own way to gain entrance into a medical convention which was held in Atlanta.

One of the therapies he discovered there which claimed success in sustaining cancer patients was a low dose chemotherapy approach using experimental drugs. The method was devised by a doctor in Germany, and Chuck obtained all the available literature. The doctor had a sizable following in Europe and his reputation was growing in the United States. His approach was a holistic one, combining drug therapy with relaxation techniques, positive thought patterns, and the like. But, while Chuck investigated this alternative therapy, Phyllis underwent the mastectomy which was followed up with conventional treatment.

After recuperating from her second surgery, she called me one day to ask if I had ever heard of a Father Ralph DiOrio. "Yes," I said. "He is part of the Charismatic Renewal and I know he has a healing ministry."

She had read his book *A Miracle to Proclaim* and had just recently discovered that he would be conducting a healing service at Madison Square Garden on June 30, 1984. She was curious to know what my impressions were. Unfortunately, I had never seen Fr. DiOrio, but had heard many wonderful things about him. She and Chuck were going to the service and wondered if it would be possible for Ed and me to meet them in New York.

Having suffered the severe blow of an unexpected recurrence, it was obvious that she was reaching out to God for healing. Fr. DiOrio's book was replete with personal testimonies of miraculous intervention in the lives of ordinary people. Naturally, it was understandable that she would want to pursue such a course herself. My reaction was one of cautious optimism. In fact, I told her, "Phyllis, you may walk out of Madison Square Garden with the same cancer you walked in with, but I know you will be healed in some way. God will honor your faith." I believed that then and I believe that now. She was delighted when I said we would join them and make a day of it.

The morning of the event, we met at their hotel located across the street from the Garden. Already the crowd was swelling, so we wasted no time getting into line. Once inside, we hurriedly made our way to the chairs close to the stage and placed Phyllis in an aisle seat, on the chance that Fr. DiOrio might come down among the people.

All along the perimeter people were lined up in wheelchairs. We noticed a young couple in the section directly behind us with a child who looked about three, weighed down with leg braces. There was an aisle formed in back of us separating our section from the rows behind—later we realized it would be used as an access to usher the handicapped to the stage where Fr. DiOrio would lay hands on them.

There was a row of empty chairs on the stage, and, one by one, they began to be filled by members of the clergy. The singing from the choir filled the air as we watched thousands of people pouring in on all sides of the Garden. There were over 18,000 people in attendance that day.

A hush fell over the audience as we were led in the recitation of the rosary. Each decade was interspersed with songs of praise, converting the gigantic arena into a house of prayer.

When the rosary ended, I turned to Phyllis and said, "How do you suppose two little Irish Catholic girls from Pittsburgh ever ended up at a healing service conducted by a Catholic priest in Madison Square Garden?" No sooner were the words out of my mouth when Fr. DiOrio, center stage, looked out into the vast audience and said, "How do you suppose a little Italian boy from Rhode Island ever got to Madison Square Garden conducting a healing service as a Catholic priest?" Astonished, Phyllis did a double take that would put Groucho Marx to shame. I just shrugged my shoulders and shook my head in wonder. It was so crazy, we both broke into gales of laughter.

Laughter is good for the soul and, in addition to our hopes and prayers, we shared a great deal of laughter that day. We needed to laugh because there was so much at stake, and we were all so tense. I've always maintained that God has a wonderful sense of humor, and I'm sure He did not think us irreverent when Chuck glanced sideways, cast his eyes on my husband's somewhat sparse hairline and exclaimed, "I do believe I see more hair growing on your head!" His timing was superb—it was just what we needed to loosen up and relax.

Fr. DiOrio asked the audience to remain in their seats. Obviously, it was impossible for everyone present to go to him, so only those in wheelchairs were to be brought to the front. He stressed the fact that God would be touching many people and He would heal them right where they were seated.

After calling us to repentance and prayer, designated escorts began to form lines leading the handicapped to the stage. The young man behind us lifted the child with leg braces into his arms and carried him forward. We sat in silent wonder as we watched the parade of wheelchairs slowly making their way to the front of the stadium.

Fr. DiOrio gently and respectfully prayed over each one. A number of people were so awestruck with the reality of God's presence at that moment that their bodies became limp and they "rested in the Spirit." Resting in the Spirit can last for a few moments or several hours. It happened to me once while I was being prayed over: I was completely conscious but, at the same time, overcome with an inner peace that rendered all around me insignificant. All my fears, all anxieties were replaced by my awareness of God's love. Resting in the Spirit is like a physical embrace from the Lord.

Many removed their braces before making their way back to their seats. The young man returned to his seat behind us cradling the little boy in one arm and holding the leg braces in the other. We all witnessed this tiny child taking small steps entirely on his own. He didn't run or jump, but he *was* trying to walk without the braces. Phyllis and I both noticed the young mother of this child—from the look of frustration and anguish on her face, it was obvious that she was unable to accept these tentative steps as a prelude to healing. Eventually she placed the braces back on the child's legs. On seeing this, a woman sitting directly in front of us sighed, "She shouldn't do that—she is denying God's healing power."

This statement was a serious challenge to my faith. Would I, in similar circumstances, have enough trust in God to step out in faith? Or would I be fainthearted, play it safe, and return the braces to the child? It was a question I could not honestly answer. I had no doubt that all healing comes from God, but how effective can our prayers be, I wondered, if we do not truly yield ourselves to be used as instruments through which He can work? Phyllis and I glanced at one another, both pondering the mystery in our own silence.

Fr. DiOrio was gathering a number of people on stage. One man, a member of the clergy, excitedly proclaimed that God had restored his hearing. One by one, each person on that stage shared his or her miraculous healing with the audience. This was the Gospel alive in a way I had never before experienced. In all candor, my faith was probably smaller than a mustard seed, yet I recognized that what I saw and heard that day had to be a display of God's power. Christ promised that the blind would see and the lame would walk.

The service lasted over five hours, but we felt no weariness; it was as if time were suspended. Everything flowed so gracefully—a sure sign of the Holy Spirit's presence. I never before experienced such a communion of hearts and minds, all united in the common belief of the power of Jesus Christ!

I had attended only one healing service before in my life and it was small in comparison. I wasn't sure what to expect at a service of such magnitude. There is always the possibility of a carnival atmosphere in any healing service— the danger often lies in the excessive emotionalism of the participants. In our Catholic faith, the apostolic gift of "laying on of hands" has been practiced for centuries; it is just recently, however, that healing services have become widespread. Many Catholics are not only unfamiliar with this ministry, but they would probably greet it with skepticism. Fr. DiOrio clarified all my doubts—his doctrine was sound and his style engaging.

After the service, we found a small intimate restaurant where we rehashed the day's events. Chuck told us that he knew their fate was in God's hands, but he still felt a responsibility to explore every possible angle. Actually, despite the gravity of their situation, we spent very little time in serious conversation—we were too busy enjoying each other's company. Patrons in the restaurant who saw us talking and laughing would have found it impossible to believe that Phyllis had a catastrophic illness.

We wanted to savor every minute of this time together, but unfortunately the hour was late and they had a plane to catch. Ed and I drove them to the airport and while *we* would return to our daily routine, such a luxury was not available to our friends.

After the Madison Square Garden experience, I found myself fantasizing that Phyllis would be cured. She would be one more "miracle to proclaim," I thought. How amazed her doctors would be when they found no evidence of cancer! My expectations were so strong, I couldn't bring myself to call her, afraid of what she might tell me. Finally, at the end of July, curiosity overwhelmed me and I phoned. It was a bitter disappointment: physically, nothing had changed, and emotionally she was consumed with fear.

The Visit

...He guides me in right paths
for His name's sake.
Psalm 23:3

In an effort to learn more about the widely-acclaimed experimental treatment from Germany, Phyllis and Chuck made an appointment to see a doctor in New York who was an advocate of this method of therapy. Eventually, they hoped to travel to Germany to meet the doctor who had devised the therapy, but the waiting list was long. They took a plane to New York the night before their appointment and returned home the next day; to my disappointment, there was not enough time for us to get together.

By this time, we were communicating on a weekly basis, sometimes more often. So when I spoke with Phyllis after the trip to New York, she told me that it was informative, but posed a problem for her. She described the holistic approach they encouraged. Tired and confused but, more than anything, apprehensive, she asked me if I knew what "dowsing" meant.

"I've never heard of such a thing," I confessed.

"Well," she explained, "we've been in touch with some of the people named in their literature, and one of them told us we might possibly need a dowser—a person who locates geopathic zones in your household in an effort to dispel oppressive forces!"

From the terminology they used, it sounded to me like psychic healing. Although she was so vulnerable, so eager for answers, Phyllis knew instinctively this was potentially dangerous. "Marion, it's hard enough dealing with the cancer, but this! We're dealing with my immortal soul."

She asked me if I knew of anyone who might be familiar with such methods. Suddenly I remembered a man from my prayer group, Larry, who was involved in the healing ministry. He had a great deal of experience and I thought perhaps he could provide some answers. As soon as I finished talking to Phyllis, I called him and explained the problem. I was relieved to learn that he knew exactly what a dowser was.

"It can be found in Scripture, in the Old Testament," he said. "Dowsing comes from the family of divination—the use of spirits to gain knowledge and information. It was expressly forbidden by Moses." (Dt. 18:10)

He then asked if I thought Phyllis might consider coming to New Jersey. "I would be most happy to counsel and pray for your friend."

My immediate response was, "She's already been to a Father DiOrio healing service!" Then, embarrassed by my outburst, I hastily apologized. "Forgive me, Larry, you know a prophet is never recognized in his own home town!" Fortunately, he had a good sense of humor about my comment and showed nothing but sincerity and compassion towards Phyllis's problem.

"After all," he went on, "you did say she was seriously considering a trip to Germany if and when she could get an appointment. If she is willing to travel that far, why not ask her to come here?"

It certainly made sense to me, so I told him I would extend the offer. At first, Phyllis seemed to have reservations, however, she agreed to give the idea some thought and get back to me. Surprisingly, the next evening she called to say she was coming. Her only concern had been leaving her younger son, but shortly after our conversation, he was asked to join his aunt and uncle for a week at the shore. This unexpected invitation meant she would be free to travel. She immediately made arrangements to fly into Newark airport on the following Tuesday, July 31. I remember the date vividly because it was the night before my baby Katie's birthday. I never mentioned this fact to Phyllis. Knowing her as I did, she would have refused to come, thinking this an imposition.

Having extended this invitation, I was a little more than anxious. Her trip to Madison Square Garden had not brought about a miracle; what was to be gained in coming to New Jersey? I knew I should trust and rely on the Lord, but in reality I was afraid of creating a false hope—or promising her more than I could deliver.

A birthday party had already been scheduled, for Katie's birthday is a very special occasion in our house. She had come to us very late in life and most unexpectedly; her presence in our lives is a constant reminder of God's love. Katie was indeed a miracle, and Phyllis knew every detail surrounding her birth.

My husband and I have a blood incompatibility which had resulted in the loss of three children. It was a progressive and irreversible problem, and when I discovered at the age of forty-three that I was pregnant, my heart was filled with despair. There was no hope for this child, but, I tried to tell myself, with God all things are possible. I prayed and hoped for a miracle, and God answered my plea. Even the medical experts were in awe at her survival. She was born on August 1, 1980 and is now a beautiful, precocious child. It's easy to understand, therefore, why her birthday has a significance which transcends the ordinary joy of a family celebration.

All the children invited to the party belonged to friends in my prayer group. Balloons of every shade, attached to crepe paper birthday streamers, festooned the trees in the backyard. The picnic table was covered with party decorations.

"God love them," Phyllis said, watching their innocent faces as they squealed with laughter, playing tag among the trees. My sixteen year old daughter supervised the festivities in the back yard while Phyllis and I and three friends sat and shared stories all afternoon.

Nothing had been planned ahead, but this spontaneous get-together brought out story after story of God's powerful touch in the lives of those present. I could see Phyllis absorbing each detail. She was so full of questions, wanting to know how each of us had experienced this need, this hunger that only God can satisfy. Each woman shared her own experience of the unique way in which God had called her into a deeper, more personal walk with Him.

Phyllis told all of us how much she wished she had what we had. Tears welled up in her eyes as she told how frightened she was, how unable to concentrate on even the smallest matter. Cancer can cripple the mind of its victims, and she so desperately wanted to be able to relax. Her outward appearance certainly belied the inner terror which was controlling her. She described the fear as paralyzing—it consumed her night and day.

Phyllis told us how she had experienced a baptism in the Holy Spirit but, she sighed, "It was years ago and I don't think it took." The women at the table laughed knowingly at these familiar and humble words. She went on to explain, however, that she did not follow through by joining a prayer community and consequently had no support.

We assured her that day of how much God loved and cared for her. She had only to believe and respond to His perfect love. We explained how so often we can accept God's love in an academic way but stop short of drawing closer, afraid of what that might mean; knowing God's love intellectually is a poor substitute for experiencing it with our whole being. This informal sharing was more than a blessing—it set the stage for what was to come.

That evening Phyllis and I went to Larry's home. When

we arrived, Larry's wife, Vada, a very kind and gracious lady, extended a warm welcome to each of us. I was pleasantly surprised to discover that Michael, a young man from our parish, was there. I had first met Michael, a recent convert, at a prayer meeting. He had not been baptized as a child, yet he responded to the Lord's call beautifully. Hungry for answers, he attended the "Life in the Spirit" seminars in our parish. At about the same time, he participated in the RCIA program (Rite of Christian Initiation of Adults), after which he received the sacraments of Baptism, Penance, Holy Eucharist, and Confirmation.

Baptism in the Holy Spirit was the culmination of an already fantastic year for Michael. He fell in love with Scripture and was rarely seen without his Bible. God lavished powerful gifts on him, but he was particularly drawn to the healing ministry and begged the Lord to use him in some way. His prayers were answered and, before long, he found himself ministering to, praying for, and consoling the many souls God put in his path.

All day I had found myself imagining this moment, and for some reason, I kept thinking, "Wouldn't it be nice if Michael were there!" How thoughtful it was of Larry to include him.

Also present was a woman from the neighboring Episcopal church who had come, at Larry's invitation, to join in prayer for Phyllis. She was introduced to me as Nance Mellon, and while we had never met before, her name had come up frequently in conversation with others I knew. Everyone's presence there was a blessed assurance to me. I knew this was going to be very special.

We were led by Larry into the prayer room, a room set aside in their home just for the Lord. How very beautiful! Just as a meticulously adorned table enhances a meal, so too a special prayer room sets the tone for communicating with our Lord. A light beige couch was against one wall, and centered above it was an impressive charcoal drawing of Christ crucified, framed in natural wood. Against the wall to the left of the couch stood a small mahogany cabinet which had a small, delicate pedestal attached to the back of it. A votive light placed atop the pedestal shone directly on a crucifix nailed to the wall. A white cloth was draped over the cabinet and a beautifully carved wooden chalice was positioned in the center. There were other articles on the cabinet: a rosary, a vial of blessed oil, and a bottle of holy water.

We sat on the couch, facing a large bookcase. My eyes were drawn to the number of books Larry had, and I hastily tried to read the titles. There were several translations of the Bible, some scholarly theological treatises, biographies of the saints, books on divine healing, and a variety of meditation books. It was a spiritual treasure chest.

We didn't know what to expect, but Nance put us at ease immediately with her own remarkable story of a miraculous healing from cancer. Seven years ago, she told us, she lay dying in a hospital room. She, too, had breast cancer, and everything medically possible had been done for her. Nance frankly admitted that during her illness she had no great faith in God and, therefore, put her faith in the doctor. The only thing she was certain of was her desire to live. But she continued to deteriorate. Finally, realizing her helplessness, she called out to God and said, "Either take me, or take me and use me."

At that moment, she knew that God had healed her. According to Nance, there was no physical evidence of a cure then or for a long time afterwards, yet there was no doubt in her mind that God had touched her. More important than her physical healing was the spiritual conversion Nance experienced. It was this conversion that led her into the healing ministry.

Phyllis and I were both enthralled with this story. I can think of nothing that gives more hope than a personal witness of God's action in one's life. Phyllis then told us all how nervous and frightened she was. She explained her present situation, including the fact that she was exploring every medical avenue that might provide an answer.

Although I was not part of the healing ministry, I was invited to join the others in prayer. It was quite a moving experience for me—they came before God with such simplicity, sincerity, and childlike trust. Nance raised her voice in song, praying in tongues. This special gift from the Holy Spirit is especially beneficial when our own words fail us. It is often referred to as praying in the Spirit (1 Cor. 14:14-15).

In the silence of my heart, I asked God to protect Phyllis. She was so vulnerable. It would have been easier for me to join in prayer for a stranger; with my close friend, there was this underlying anxiety of "what if she isn't healed?" as if a miracle depended upon me and my performance and not on God.

It was still early in the evening when they finished and I suggested to Phyllis that we go to a prayer meeting. The meetings are held in the cafeteria of our parish grade school which is a very large room. Sometimes our group looks lost in a room that size, but this night it was packed. I craned my neck looking for all my close friends, especially those women who had met Phyllis earlier in the afternoon at the birthday party. One of them, Kathy, was missing, and I was so disappointed. This was a special occasion and I wanted to share it with the people who had come to mean so much to me in my spiritual journey. Kathy not only inspired me by her personal example, but also took the time to help me in every way possible to grow in God's grace. To my surprise and delight, she walked in later, all dressed up with a beautiful red rose pinned on the lapel of her jacket. She told me later that she had no intention of missing this prayer meeting, but a dinner engagement had run a little late.

It's interesting to note that I had never met Kathy before entering the prayer community. But she was the one I turned to with countless questions on Catholicism and renewal, and her common sense and wisdom were invaluable. We were both "POFs" (parents over forty), and this established a mutual affinity immediately. Added to that, we soon discovered we had both been born and raised in Pittsburgh and even knew some of the same people; yet our paths had never crossed. We think we choose our own friends, but I believe that, in this instance God laid out a friendship for me. This was brought clearly into focus for me after I had known Kathy for about three years.

My mother had come to live with me, and one day, rummaging through a box of her old photos, I came across a picture of my cousin at her high school graduation. Standing next to her was a girl who looked very familiar. To my complete astonishment, it turned out to be none other than my new friend, Kathy. I found out later that Kathy's sister graduated in the same class and whoever snapped the picture caught her beside my cousin. At the time I thought to myself that this was another loving touch from God—nothing overwhelming, just a simple and gentle reminder that He is truly interested in every aspect of our lives.

Because the room was so crowded, the leader asked that prayer requests be kept until the end of the meeting at which time we would offer up a general petition to cover everyone's needs. Phyllis blushed in embarrassment as I bolted out of my seat and exclaimed that I certainly didn't want to upset the applecart, but I had a specific request. I looked around the room and explained to all there that this was my friend from Pittsburgh whom they had been praying for over the past year. "I brought her here tonight for one reason—that all of you might join together and ask for God's healing."

Everyone present responded in a visible way. Some waved, others smiled and nodded, several came over and warmly embraced Phyllis, welcoming her to our meeting. A chair was placed in the center of the room for Phyllis to sit in while everyone united in prayer, asking God to touch and heal this beautiful woman for whom they had prayed so faithfully before even meeting her.

Phyllis was so shy, yet so grateful for this prayer. She sat quietly in the chair, her hands tightly clasped. It was Kathy who approached her and asked, "Would you like a new infilling of the Holy Spirit?"

Answering softly, yet earnestly, she replied, "Yes, I would."

"Lord, I ask you to send down your Holy Spirit to fill her."

With piety and humility, Phyllis tried to whisper the words in unison. Resting her hand on Phyllis's shoulder, Kathy continued to pray, "Lord, please draw her closer to you." Here Phyllis's words became audible, "And even if I am not healed, dear Jesus, I want you to come into my life."

There was a lovely smile on her lips after this prayer, and her body assumed a posture of total relaxation, full of peace. We then joined hands in thanksgiving and it was exhilarating to watch all the joyful faces. I felt as though I was an honored guest at a marvelous party where everyone was having a wonderful time.

My friend Elvira, who had been at my home earlier that afternoon, walked over to me looking radiant and said, "Marion, do you realize what day this is?" I knew immediately what she meant by the significance of this particular day—it was a day for miracles. Because it was the day of my Katie's birth, it gave me great hope, that if God had spared Katie, maybe he would spare Phyllis as well.

Just before we left, Kathy asked Phyllis if she knew

anyone in Pittsburgh who belonged to a prayer community.

"As a matter of fact, I do. There is an old friend, Sally, a girl Marion and I went to school with, who has been taking me to prayer meetings at St. Thomas More Church."

What a pleasant coincidence—that was the very prayer group Kathy's sister belonged to in Pittsburgh! She gave Phyllis her sister's telephone number and encouraged her to call.

As we pulled up in front of my house, Phyllis and I sat in the car reminiscing over the details of an altogether wonderful day. Truly, this was a day the Lord had made and we had ample reason to rejoice.

"Marion, I never felt so much love in one room in my whole life," she sighed. Somewhat overwhelmed, I blurted, "I can't believe what you just said! Oh, Phyllis, this is exciting!" And then I explained that several months before, our prayer group had been given a prophecy: "Whenever someone comes into your midst and feels the love, you will see miracles!"

The expression on her face changed dramatically. Her mouth dropped open, her eyebrows raised, and those intensely blue eyes began to moisten. Words were unnecessary—we could read each other's thoughts as we sat quietly in hopeful expectation. After a few moments of silence, Phyllis smiled and said, "I felt a warmth stirring deep inside when Kathy walked in late with that rose pinned to her jacket. It was as if I could hear Daddy's voice. He always called me his 'Little Rose.' Mother and Dad are both in my thoughts so frequently since I became ill." I thought it was interesting how a seemingly insignificant thing, under the right circumstances, can trigger an important memory.

Then she extended her arm and held out her hand. "Maybe you didn't notice, but I was so frightened before I came here I had no control over my trembling hands." Didn't notice? It was the first thing that had struck me about her! Now she sat poised and relaxed, with her hands resting gracefully in her lap.

I was beginning to recognize the tender and loving work of the Holy Spirit in all of this. It was more than I could have imagined—these personal nuances, each with their own special meaning. Prayer was opening our eyes to a glimpse of the supernatural—bringing spiritual realities into our world in a way we could and would recognize.

Phyllis wanted to spend the following day with her sister Ann. They made arrangements to meet for lunch at a shopping center close to my home. After greeting each other enthusiastically with hugs and kisses, Ann held her baby sister at arm's length and with a playful grin announced, "You and I are going to visit a dear friend in Philadelphia!"

A puzzled Phyllis smiled, wondering aloud who it was they knew in Philadelphia.

"The man himself—St. John Neumann," replied Ann. "I'm taking you to the church where he is buried."

How kind and thoughtful of Ann to think of such an outing. From the beginning of her illness, the relic of St. John Neumann had never been far from Phyllis, and she continued to rely on his intercession.

I left the two sisters and got into my car, thanking God with all my heart for this very special visit. Everything was falling into place so well. If I had planned each step (which I hadn't), it would never have flowed so perfectly. Truthfully, once I knew that Phyllis was actually coming, I was very anxious and worried, but Kathy told me not to worry what might or might not happen: I had done my part by extending the invitation—the rest was up to the Holy Spirit.

"But Kathy," I insisted, "this is one of my dearest and oldest friends. What if..." Once again, she gave me the assurance that God would handle the situation—all I had to do was trust Him. It was true. I could see it happening.

In the early evening, a beaming Phyllis returned and told me it had been another perfectly wonderful day. When they arrived at St. Peter's in Philadelphia, the church was empty, save for the janitor. He was kind enough to escort them to the area where St. John Neumann was buried, and he allowed both of them to hold the chalice which belonged to this revered saint. This was a gratifying experience for Phyllis—a chance to connect personally with a saint she knew only from afar. How gracious of our Lord to arrange for such a private meeting.

As soon as she freshened up, we went back to Larry and Vada's house. We were delighted to see that Michael was there again. These three wonderful people have no extraordinary power of their own (so many people harbor false notions about the healing ministry); I'm convinced God uses them as channels in the healing gifts because of their childlike obedience and trust in Him. It is by their honest and sincere prayers that the power of Jesus is often revealed. He promised that when two or more were gathered in His name, He would be there.

After praying for some time, we sat back in quiet reflection. Phyllis, with the wide-eyed innocence of a child broke the silence. "What do you think I should do—I mean, how should I proceed when I get back home?"

Larry, squatting comfortably on the plush carpet, stretched his legs. "I encourage you to have faith in your doctors," he said without hesitation.

"But the dowser! What about that?"

He broke into a wide grin as he said, "Pray, with complete honesty. Go before the Lord. He will protect you from all harm and remove any deterrent to your spiritual welfare, including a dowser!"

Vada and Michael echoed their agreement. It was all so simple. "Oh ye of little faith" I murmured to myself.

I held a great fascination for the healing ministry and had read several books on the subject, written by people with impeccable credentials. However, this was the first opportunity I had to personally talk to individuals intimately involved in the ministry. I couldn't resist asking Larry the obvious question, "Have all the people you prayed for been cured?"

With a broad smile, Larry answered, "When you've been involved in the healing ministry for any length of time, you acknowledge that God's perfect healing is death." But he hastened to add, "Now, Phyllis, I want very much for you to live and I will continue to pray for a complete cure. I'm only saying our faith teaches us that God perfects us in our death."

This was startling to me—it was something I had never really thought about. I then wondered how it was possible to go on—to pray for healing when no change is apparent.

"Were you ever disappointed?" I asked.

The question most definitely touched a raw nerve. Larry stared right into my eyes as he said, "Oh yes—I've even been angry! It concerned a man I prayed for who was critically ill and in a coma. I was part of a healing team, and we prayed every night for two weeks for this man. Suddenly he began to show signs of recognition, especially when his wife entered the room. Even the doctors thought something was happening, and they increased his caloric intake. And, then, without warning, the man developed pneumonia and died!

"I just couldn't understand why," Larry continued. "Before we prayed, the man's wife had accepted the fact he was going to die, but when he began to rally, she was certain he would live. I was angry with the Lord—it made no sense to me. Then, one day, I was on my way into a store when I heard a car horn toot. A man called me over and asked if I remembered him.

" 'No, I'm afraid not,' I replied.

"The man said, 'I saw you pray for my friend when he was dying in the hospital. It's the first time I can honestly say I saw people who could be described as true Christians. I just want you to know that I hadn't been to church in years but I'm back now, thanks to you and your example!'

"This was a most important lesson to me about the divine plan," Larry said. "God brings goodness out of every situation where prayer is involved."

What a beautiful example of our Lord's kindness in removing anxiety, I thought to myself.

Before we left, Larry embraced Phyllis warmly and declared, "Now it is your time to receive gifts." She didn't know what that meant, nor for that matter did he. Sometimes the Holy Spirit inspires us to say things when we have no clear understanding of the depth of our words.

The Book

I will give you treasure out of the
darkness, and riches that have been
hidden away....
Isaiah 45:3

As soon as we got home from Larry's, I put on a pot of
coffee while Phyllis slipped out of her shoes and drew her
feet up on the couch. She was refreshed and happy and so
animated that she kept up a running conversation between
sips of coffee. All at once she became very still—something
had obviously distracted her. With an expression of great
surprise, she reached down and picked up a book of mine,
He and I,* that was sitting on the table in front of us.

"Where did you get this?" she asked incredulously.
Before I could answer, she continued, "Marion, I take this
book with me everywhere I go. In fact, it's back in my
suitcase right now!"

"You're kidding!" I exclaimed.

"No," she said. "A friend of ours gave me a copy a few
years ago while we were vacationing in California. It has
become my constant companion."

"Actually, Phyllis, the way it came into my possession
was an answer to a prayer."

"What do you mean?" she asked.

I welcomed the chance to share with her the wonderful
way the book was brought to my attention. I was just an
"infant" in the Charismatic Renewal filled with excitement

* *He and I* is available from St. Bede's Publications

at my growing knowledge of the Holy Spirit. But although the Renewal was opening my eyes to a better understanding of the Holy Spirit, I had all but forgotten Mary and her role as our Mother. One day, on my knees scrubbing the kitchen floor, I told the Lord how confused I was about her. (I find that my most profound answers to prayer usually come when I'm involved in the most humble of circumstances.) I asked Him very simply, "Where does Mary fit in, Lord?" This small but honest question brought about remarkable results.

The following week at a Pro Life National Convention, I met a woman with whom I struck up a conversation, and after a while, she asked me if I was a Charismatic. "Yes I am," I said. "And how exciting it is to be part of the Renewal and see firsthand what God is doing for His people. One thing troubles me though—in all my new-found joy, I've been thinking a lot about the Blessed Mother, wondering just where she fits into God's plan."

The woman smiled as if she had expected my comment. "I have a book you might like to read. It will put everything in its proper perspective," she assured me. Naturally, I was intrigued. She hurried off to her room, and minutes later, this kind stranger handed me her copy of *He and I*. She graciously suggested that I take it home and read it at my leisure.

Never before had I been so emotionally touched by a book. In fact, I wouldn't part with it until I had bought a copy for myself.

He and I is a living book that speaks to one's heart and touches the depths of the soul. Originally comprising two separate volumes, it is now available in one book. The first volume of *He and I* was published anonymously in 1948, and even the author's closest friends did not know that she was the author. It was only after her death and the publication of the second volume that her identity was revealed.

It is the diary of a French woman, Gabrielle Bossis, who

had a secret life in Christ, and she carefully recorded the words Jesus spoke to her every day. She was an artistic and sophisticated woman who, late in life, discovered she had a talent for writing. She began to write moral comedies which were much in demand. Her first effort was highly successful, and soon she became known throughout France. For the rest of her life, she traveled extensively, not only writing plays, but producing and acting in them as well.

The messages in her diary are universal. They are very personal to Gabrielle, yet the miracle is that these captivating conversations are just as personal to me and to all who read the book. God has spoken to me many times from the pages of this moving diary and I have no doubt He will continue to do so. I have read it from cover to cover three times, and it still blesses me.

The fact that I had this book meant a great deal to Phyllis. It was another bond between us. In discussing the book, we discovered that our commitment to the spiritual strength of this gem compelled both of us to send copies to people we knew would read it and be blessed. The irony is that passing *He and I* on to others was a gesture Phyllis accomplished even in death.

During the period when our mutual friend, Sally, took her to prayer meetings at St. Thomas More Church in Pittsburgh, Phyllis gave her the book as a gift. Sally read from it daily and experienced the same powerful attachment to it that Phyllis and I had. And, like us, she began to give copies away.

The week before Phyllis went to the hospital for the last time, Sally visited her at home and, among other things, told her how she loved *He and I*. Raising her head from the pillow, Phyllis said, "That reminds me, I've ordered four copies and I can't remember now who I wanted them for—will you pick up my order and give them away?"

"Of course I will," Sally promised.

A few days later, Sally picked up the books. She already had two people in mind, but with no clear idea about who should receive the other copies, she placed them in the glove compartment of her car.

Something quite unexpected and very comforting happened after the funeral. When the family and close friends were invited to a luncheon, Sally found herself sitting next to Phyllis's sister Rita who lives in Texas. In their conversation, Rita spoke about a book—she couldn't remember the title, but Phyllis had raved about it constantly. "As a matter of fact, she promised to send me a copy but never did."

"Don't move!" Sally told her. "I have a delightful surprise for you!"

In a matter of minutes, she was out to the car and back. Out of breath but elated, she placed the book in Rita's hands. "This book was the last thing Phyllis and I discussed. I know she intended it for you and I am so honored to be able to fulfill this one last favor for her!"

Rita was speechless as she lovingly pressed the book to her heart.

Moments later, Sally was introduced to Rita's daughter, a lovely young woman named Molly. Still glowing, Sally related the happy coincidence to Molly and something in the girl's expression prompted her to ask, "Would you like to have a copy of your own?" Molly's face lit up. "I have nothing belonging to my Aunt Phyllis—I would love to have that book!"

With her mission accomplished, a joyful Sally ran over to me to explain what had happened. "I just know Phyllis is smiling down on me at this moment!" she said happily.

Sally was certain that somehow Phyllis knew what had just taken place—and so was I!

The Promise

The promises of the Lord are sure,
like tried silver...
Psalm 12:7

The same night we discovered our mutual devotion to *He
and I,* Phyllis made another discovery. Taped on the inside
cover of my book, she noticed a small holy card with the
picture of a little girl cradled in a large hand, with the
caption: "See! I will not forget you...I have carved you on
the palm of my hand." The quotation comes from Isaiah
49:15. Phyllis kept fingering the card, studying the inscrip-
tion. Finally, she said, "I have never seen a card like this
before, Marion—where did you get it?"

"That card is a reminder to me—a memento of words the
Lord gave me at a time in my life when I desperately needed
to hear them."

Puzzled, she asked me to elaborate.

It happened, I told her, when I was going through a most
unhappy time in my life. In the midst of a deep depression, I
felt so alone; all my efforts to find consolation seemed
futile. Then, one day, in great anguish, I agreed to be
prayed over by a couple of friends. After fervent prayer,
one of these dear people gave me that message—the passage from Isaiah—telling me it was from the Lord. While
they were beautiful words and I wanted to believe they
were intended for me personally, I wasn't convinced until
they were subsequently confirmed to me three times, in
three different places and under three different circumstances.

I told Phyllis where the final, and by far the most dramatic, confirmation of those words came to me. It happened in a high school in Philadelphia, a place I had never been before. Ed and I were there attending a program as guests of friends. While standing in the lobby, waiting for the auditorium to open, I gazed around at the old structure. It was the kind no one can afford to build these days. The lobby walls were covered in pale, pinkish-gray marble from floor to ceiling. While I was surveying the height of the ceiling, I noticed there were some words carved in the marble on the wall. The message jumped out at me, worded exactly as it had been given to me when my friends prayed over me. My skepticism evaporated and I realized that our Lord does indeed communicate with us.

This confirmation dispelled my doubts, enabling me to discern His voice from my own wishful thinking. Perhaps the more mature Christian recognizes God's touch immediately, but, as for me, I needed reinforcement, and, thank God, it was, and continues to be, there.

After telling my story, Phyllis looked at me with amazement and sighed, "Oh, Marion, if only something like that would happen to me . . . . " With intensity, I assured her, "It will Phyllis, it will!"

The next day, however, feeling somewhat doubtful and questioning the authority I had spoken with, I kiddingly asked the Lord not to make a liar out of me. Phyllis was like a sponge, so spiritually thirsty, and I didn't want to be dishing out pleasant platitudes just to make her feel good.

Friday came all too soon and she had to catch an early afternoon plane back to Pittsburgh. Even though her visit was brief, much had been accomplished. So many lives were affected in large and small ways, all because she had come to New Jersey.

I asked Kathy to accompany us to the airport and she agreed to join us on the long ride up the turnpike to Newark. We began our trip by reciting the rosary together—

it seemed only fitting to end the visit on a hopeful note and, by God's grace, I had come to recognize that the rosary is a powerful prayer. My renewed devotion was most certainly a result of that small question I had asked from the kitchen floor when the Lord gently taught me what I had all but forgotten about Mary's role as intercessor.

In the short time of her visit, Phyllis had built up a strong attachment to the people from the prayer community. I could now sense her apprehension about leaving as she sighed, "If only I could take all of you back to Pittsburgh." It was flattering to hear, but Kathy and I told her that it was the prayers that mattered, not the people, and we promised that we would continue to storm heaven for her.

Phyllis only had one small suitcase, so we dropped her off right outside the ticket counter. She kissed Kathy on the cheek and promised once again to contact her sister in Pittsburgh. Then, giving me a big bear hug, she promised she would be in touch soon. Kathy and I got back into the car and watched her until she disappeared from sight.

Driving home, I told Kathy how foolish my anxiety had been about the visit. Everything had gone perfectly. It reminded me of the words from a song, "Every little movement has a meaning all its own." All that had happened during her stay had to have been orchestrated by the Holy Spirit. Every gesture, every word was hand-tailored to minister to Phyllis where she needed it most. I will always be grateful for such a marvelous experience which was made possible by God's divine love.

The following Wednesday, at the prayer meeting, I told everyone that Phyllis said she had never felt so much love in one room as she did the night she was with us. When I reminded them of the prophecy we had received—that when someone could feel the love in our midst, we would experience miracles and healing—they were visibly impressed.

Still basking in the glow of Phyllis's visit, I had to telephone Jayne, my special "guardian angel"—a term of endearment I began to use after learning that she had prayed for me before she even knew me. Because our husbands worked for the same company, she learned— although unknown to me—that my baby was in jeopardy. As the deeply devout woman she is, she pleaded with God to spare my child, and after Katie's birth, she continued to pray for me. I feel most certainly that it was her prayer that brought me back to my knees and taught me how to respond to God's love.

Knowing how faithful she would be, Jayne was the first person I had called for prayer when I found out that Phyllis had cancer. She, in turn, asked all the people in her fellowship to pray for Phyllis. Nance Mellon, who had told us at Larry's house how she had survived cancer, was part of Jayne's group—but there was no way any of us could know we would be drawn together through Phyllis. God's way of calling on different sources to accomplish His plan is truly wonderful.

During the time Phyllis was at my home, we had dropped in at Jayne's for just a few minutes. She was grateful for the opportunity to meet Phyllis, if only briefly, and like everyone else, was struck by her beauty.

Now, on the phone, she said, "It's so good to be able to put a face with the name when we're called to pray for someone." I replied, "I'm only sorry we didn't have more time to spend with you, Jayne. The visit was a great success—everything flowed in perfect harmony and, believe me, I had no game plan!"

"God's itinerary is always perfect!" Jayne rejoiced. She went on, "I have something special to share with you that concerns Phyllis. Nance told me that before going to Larry's home that night, she called an Episcopalian priest we both know. Along with others in our fellowship, this priest is part of the Order of St. Luke, a healing ministry under the auspices of the Episcopal Church. She wanted him to

back her up in prayer so that she might minister success-
fully to Phyllis. He not only agreed, but immediately went
into the chapel, and, knowing Phyllis was a Catholic, lit a
candle and prayed for her himself."

"Nance's contribution that night at Larry's was a special
bonus," I said. "Her own battle and miraculous deliverance
from cancer were an inspiration to Phyllis. And the fact
that she devotes her life as a healing vessel for others was
an inspiration to me!"

Jayne added, "Nance's witness is a perfect illustration
that God hears our prayers." She was right—the prayers
were important and we both agreed to continue even more
vigorously.

*   *   *

To think all these wonderful people were right in my
own back yard all this time. Just a few short years ago, I
knew nothing about a personal relationship with Jesus or
the power of the Holy Spirit, nor did I know people who
had experienced this new life. When the Holy Spirit
empowers us, He gives us the grace and vision to recognize
God's action in our lives. It's still exciting to me in my own
spiritual odyssey that the right people just seem to find
each other at the right moment. Even more exciting is the
generosity of our Lord in sending so many people who
would become involved in the life of my precious friend.

I had a taste of things to come that first night at Larry's
home. While we were there, Nance told Phyllis her son
lived in Pittsburgh and she just happened to be going to
visit him the very next week. "Would you like me to come
to see you at that time?" she asked.

"Oh, please do!" Phyllis responded.

Such concern and compassion after one meeting can
only come from God.

The Statue

See! I will not forget you...I have
carved you on the palm of my hand.
Isaiah 49:15

On a Sunday afternoon, exactly nine days after visiting
me, Phyllis called from Pittsburgh, her voice breathless
with excitement. "Marion, I have some wonderful news—
are you sitting down?" I wasn't, but I promptly did so. She
continued, "Do you remember Larry telling me before I
left his home that it was my time to receive gifts?"

"Yes, I remember."

She then told me that that very morning her husband,
Chuck, and their son, Mark, went to an early Mass, and she
decided to take her other son, Kevin, to the noon Mass in a
neighboring parish. When they arrived, she saw all sorts of
people in the back of the church, people with obvious signs
of illness, some even in wheelchairs. A woman with a red
corsage pinned on her dress gave Phyllis a warm smile.
Curious, she asked, "Is this a Mass where they bless the
sick?" "Yes it is," the woman whispered. When Phyllis
asked who was in charge, the woman pointed to a nun who
was standing by the side door busily coordinating everything.

"Marion, you know how shy I am, but I walked right up
to Sister and asked if I could receive the sacrament of the
sick. She seemed rather puzzled and after some hesitation,
she said, 'What's wrong with you?' I told her 'I have cancer,
Sister.'

"With that, she wrote my name on the bottom of her list,

pinned a carnation on my dress, and ushered me to a seat in the last pew. I knelt down and, looking up at the altar, my eyes were drawn to a large silver tray, placed on a table adjacent to the altar. It was filled with packages, all different sizes and shapes, beautifully wrapped with ribbons. At the beginning of Mass, the priest came down from the altar and anointed all of the sick. After communion, he came down the aisle again, this time laden with those packages I had seen. I thought I should explain to him that I had come in uninvited, but before I could say anything, he selected a present from the tray and handed it to me. I thanked him as graciously as I could, and when we got into the car to go home, I asked Kevin to open it for me.

"Marion, I couldn't believe what I saw. Inside the box was a ceramic statue of the 'Hand' cradling a little girl. At its base were the words: *See! I will not forget you . . . I have carved you on the palm of my hand.* Poor Kevin, he had no idea why I was crying and I couldn't explain. I was so overwhelmed I couldn't even speak! Marion, you told me that I would experience a confirmation from God—don't you remember?"

Drawing a deep breath, I sat in silent awe. Never could I have dreamed up such a perfect means of communication—with this extravagant gesture, God had left no room for doubt in Phyllis's mind. He had not only given her this visible sign as a keepsake, He had given His word that He would never forget her, using the identical words He had given me—words that had made such a profound impression on her.

I rejoiced with her and told her how thrilled I was for her—and for myself as well. "Can you believe the goodness of God giving you that small token just because He knew how much it would please you? You must never doubt how much He cares for you and how concerned He is about your welfare."

I could hardly wait to spread the good news of this

beautiful event. Nance Mellon actually had the opportunity to see the statue when she visited Phyllis in Pittsburgh. As soon as she got back to New Jersey, she joyfully shared the story with all those in her prayer group. My golden opportunity to tell everyone came when I went to my own prayer meeting on Wednesday night: the leader asked for one person—only one—to please give a witness that would edify the whole group. When no one else stood up, I was certain that our Lord wanted me to speak out. The room broke into loud applause—everyone was thrilled with the story of the statue.

The words from Isaiah, already indelibly etched in my own mind, had now taken on a special meaning for those who would become closely involved with Phyllis. My friend Elvira, shortly after hearing the story of the statue, had her own personal experience with regard to this same passage. It happened at a Sunday Mass: she had just received Communion and had knelt down to say a special prayer for Phyllis. She was meditating with such intensity that she was oblivious to the fact that, all around her, people were seated again. A faint echo of music in the background interrupted her concentration and she raised her head at the exact moment that the choir was singing the words: "And I will hold you in the palm of my hand!"

The Intercessors

Is there anyone sick among you?
Pray over him anointing him with
oil in the name of the Lord.
James 5:14

After hearing about the statue, I was convinced God was going to heal Phyllis physically—it was evident to me that He was responding to the outpouring of our prayers. Why, I reasoned, would He go to all the trouble of bringing her into contact with so many different people who would establish a network of prayer for her if He were not going to cure her? His grace was the only explanation for the commitment to prayer experienced by people who had just met Phyllis recently. Such an abundance of grace must have been to prepare our hearts for a miracle, I thought.

Phyllis continued to attend Monday night prayer meetings at St. Thomas More Church. I saw God's hand in that also—two prayer communities in two different states were constantly interceding on her behalf.

It was a month before I heard from her again. This time, she was frightened. She had discovered a rash near her incision and also feared there was a lump on her arm. I put out an immediate request for prayers and placed her name on the intercessory prayer line of our prayer community, a small group of devoted people who pray around the clock for special needs.

Phyllis told me that she had made an appointment to see her oncologist immediately upon discovering the lump.

The visits were such an ordeal for her; fighting the fear of the unknown sapped all her strength.

After a careful examination, her doctor told her that he would have to order more blood tests. He also said that it would be necessary to have a consultation with her surgeon who, unfortunately, would not be available for a few days. Unable to fight the stinging sensation in her eyes, she let the tears flow freely. She told me that her doctor tried to comfort her by softly patting her hand, but the only response she could manage was an aching cry, "How will I ever get through the agonizing wait?" There was nothing he could say.

At this point, Chuck decided that new steps had to be taken. "Let's pursue the experimental treatment now," he suggested. Confident that he was right, he tried to persuade a reluctant Phyllis. Her prior visit to New York had never been discussed with her Pittsburgh doctors, and she was afraid that they might discontinue treating her if they discovered she was involved, even minimally, with alternative therapies.

On the day of her appointment with the surgeon, I stopped at Larry's home, but Vada, answering the door, said he was out of town. When she asked me to come in, I stammered, "In a few minutes, Phyllis will be in the surgeon's office, and, well...I thought I'd ask Larry to pray during that time."

"Why don't you and I pray together?" she offered. Nodding, I followed her into their private sanctuary of prayer, and together we knelt down. It was clear to see that Vada was a woman accustomed to frequent intercessory prayer. Her demeanor was respectful, yet the ease with which she approached the Lord made such a deep impression on me. She spoke as a child before a loving father. I was reminded of what Jesus had said: "Let the children come...the Kingdom of God belongs to such as these" (Matthew 19:14). There wasn't a trace of self-consciousness in her. Vada was as comfortable in prayer as I might be in conversation with a close personal friend. It set an example I would not soon forget.

The following evening I called Phyllis. She was distraught, not only because of what was happening, but because a man whom she and Chuck knew quite well had died during the night from cancer. I did my best to quiet her fears. "It doesn't mean you're going to die," I protested. Oh, dear Lord, help me to help her, I cried out in my heart. "Remember, God showed you personally that He has you in the palm of His hand. How many people can say that?"

"Yes, that's true, Marion," she replied, trying to muffle the mournful sounds of weeping.

But I thanked God she couldn't see me. My own insides were beginning to crumble despite the assured tone of my voice. I cannot remember what words of strength I offered, only God knows. He inspired me with words of consolation as Phyllis reached out to me for help.

The loss of a friend from the same dread disease one is suffering from would be enough to catapult anyone into fear and indecision: should they get another opinion? should they go back to New York? She was pouring out her heart to me, looking for answers. The only advice I could offer was that perhaps she should be honest with her doctors and express her doubts and fears to them.

"I simply can't do that—not yet!" she replied. "But I'm so glad you called me tonight," she continued tearfully. "I was fighting the urge to pick up the phone to call you. It's unfair to bother you so much."

Bother me? Never, I told her. It was a privilege to have her confide in me. "What about the blood tests—and the rash?" I asked.

"I don't know the results of the blood work. As far as the rash is concerned, my surgeon gave me a topical cream to apply three times a day. At this point, he isn't worried about a recurrence. The rash seems to be along the line of the prosthesis and he told me not to wear it for a while."

"When will you know about the blood tests?"

Her voice became steadier now. Talking things out seemed to help control her fear. "He still has to consult with the oncologist. He assured me that since I've already suffered one recurrence, they would be especially vigilant."

After that, I didn't hear from her for a while. I later learned that she and Chuck had gone to their California home in Palm Springs; both of them needed a change of scenery. In the absence of any further news and because she was able to get away, I assumed the tests were all negative.

Phyllis normally called me on Wednesday evenings, the night of my prayer meetings; it was her way of reminding me not to forget her petition. When a call eventually came one Wednesday night, I was anticipating good news, but instead she made an urgent plea for prayer—after re-examining the rash, her surgeon had decided a biopsy was in order. Just the word "biopsy" sent chills through me.

I lifted her name up in petition at the prayer meeting and, afterwards, Larry, Vada, and Michael went with me into our church, which was dark and empty, and knelt down in front of the Tabernacle.

I was really too upset to pray. They asked me instead to sit in proxy for Phyllis while they knelt behind me. In the silent stillness of the church, their voices echoed in powerful prayer. Not only did they place Phyllis's needs in front of the Lord, but they asked God to bless and protect Chuck as well. I tried in vain to put myself in Phyllis's shoes, but my own anxiety made concentration impossible, so I forced myself to sit quietly, listening to their beautiful words. When they finished, we tiptoed out of the church. Blessing myself with holy water, I felt a resurgence of hope.

But Phyllis later called to tell me that the biopsy revealed some cancer cells. This news was too much for her to bear—she definitely wanted another opinion. In consulting the doctor who had examined her in New York, she learned that he did not believe the results of the biopsy: he had done elaborate blood tests on her in late October, and found no evidence of cancer. Possibly, he felt, she was having a reaction to medicine he had prescribed.

The oncologist in Pittsburgh was out of town and unavailable for consultation, so, not wanting to waste a precious moment, Phyllis and Chuck decided to follow the advice of the New York doctor. He sent them to a colleague in New Jersey—an oncologist—and treatment began immediately. The treatment was to follow the experimental procedure used in Germany, the one Chuck had first heard about at the Medical Convention.

The decision to follow this new course of treatment meant they would be traveling back and forth, staying in a motel near the doctor's office. After arrangements were made and treatment was started, Phyllis called me from the motel. Chuck had returned to Pittsburgh and she would stay on for five days.

"How would you like some company?" I asked. "Maybe some people from the prayer group will join me."

"That would be wonderful—I need their strength," she sighed.

My first impulse was to ask Larry, so I left a message with Vada. She told me that Larry would no doubt pray before agreeing to go along. Funny, I thought to myself, it had never occurred to me to pray about whom I should invite. Once again, in her gentle manner, Vada was teaching me a very important lesson—to seek God's direction in *all* things.

On my way to the prayer meeting that evening, I did pray for guidance and, with no urging on my part, both Michael and Elvira volunteered to go with me. Larry later told me he did not feel led to go along. I suspect he wanted me to realize that others could pray just as effectively as he could.

We set out the following Monday afternoon for Linden, New Jersey. Phyllis met us in the lobby of the motel, grateful for company and especially happy to see Michael and Elvira once again. Hungry from our journey, the four of us went out to dinner at a small restaurant. The meal was enjoyable, filled with light conversation and laughter. Before we finished our dessert, Phyllis unobtrusively picked up and paid the check. "You're my guests," she announced with such an air of dignity that no one dared question what she was doing. Her generous nature was no secret to me—it was her charm on such occasions that touched me.

After finishing our coffee, we walked back to the motel. Leading the way down the motel's long hallway, Phyllis stopped before one of the many identical-looking doors. But, after opening the door and turning on the light, the atmosphere suddenly and pleasantly changed. She had managed to transform an otherwise ordinary, unimpressive motel room into a lovely setting so in keeping with her character. As we stepped inside, we immediately noticed a small altar she had set up on the dresser. In the center there was a framed dedication to the Sacred Heart. There was also a statue of Mary, and off to the side was her Bible and her copy of *He and I.*

Phyllis always and everywhere afforded a place of honor to the Sacred Heart. In her own home, which was absolutely gorgeous, the main attraction of the lavishly-furnished living room was an enormous picture of the Sacred Heart of Jesus. It still hangs directly above the mantel over the fireplace, illuminated by a portrait lamp.

We didn't want to leave without praying with and for Phyllis, and, as always, she was most receptive. She lay down with her head at the foot of the bed, close to the edge. She crossed her arms over her chest and gently closed her eyes. Michael knelt on the floor near her head while Elvira and I knelt by her side. To be absolutely honest, this was an awkward moment for me, and I sensed that Elvira also was somewhat shy. We both looked to Michael, who was actively involved in the healing ministry, to lead. His youth enabled him to pray with such ease. Elvira and I, on the other hand, had to make a conscious effort to pray extemporaneously. It was difficult for us, because we had spent most of our lives thinking of prayer as a private exercise.

After a somewhat timid beginning, I found that humbling myself in this manner was a thoroughly refreshing experience. I began to realize that it wasn't necessary for us to speak eloquent and clever words. God looks at our intentions and He knows what is in our hearts. It seemed such a short time, yet the clock on the table revealed we had been on our knees for almost an hour. It was similar to my experience at Madison Square Garden—time seems to be suspended when you are spiritually unified.

We all got up, stretched our legs and settled down for a brief chat. We could have talked for hours, but it was a long trip back. "I don't know how to thank you for coming," Phyllis said affectionately, and she embraced each of us as we prepared to leave. As a parting token, she gave Elvira a copy of *He and I* and promised Michael she would send him one very soon.

Driving home, each of us individually expressed a debt of gratitude to Phyllis. Whatever trepidation we had experienced as we set out on this venture was more than compensated for by the unexpected energy and excitement we each now felt. I can only describe it as a feeling of wholeness—a fruit of the Holy Spirit after taking that step in faith.

"Isn't it wonderful?" I mused. "Here we are, three people from totally different backgrounds, bound together by a common commitment to pray for one of my oldest and dearest friends!" Certainly we hoped she would be completely cured, but for some unknown reason, I remember saying with confidence, "I have no idea what our Lord has in store for Phyllis, but one thing I am certain of—she will not leave this world a hysterical woman consumed with fear." In my mind I reflected, "Strange words for someone who believes in miracles!"

For Phyllis, the Christmas holidays added to an already stressful situation. Not being able to shop for her family upset her more than the illness itself. But the time between treatments was brief and she had to be back in New Jersey the day after Christmas.

Around the end of January, Phyllis became alarmed— her chest was inflamed and she noticed a swelling in her other breast. She called me from the motel begging for prayers. She was scheduled for a mammogram and was again the victim of that relentless fear known so well to people who suffer from cancer. Immediately, I called some personal friends and asked them to pray privately and, as always, placed her name before the prayer group. It was a great comfort knowing that so many people would eagerly and fervently respond to her need for intercession.

She was to spend the weekend with her sister Ann, and I made arrangements to drive to the motel to meet her for lunch on Monday. That weekend, for the first time, my faith began to falter—the circumstances were pretty grim. I knew realistically how bad things were, and the next morning I sat at my kitchen table sincerely asking our Lord not to look at my feelings or my confusion, but to please continue to heal Phyllis. It was as if a heavy cloud hung over me, and the validity of all the supernatural signs I myself had seen and believed was now in question.

Earnestly searching for some answer, I reached for my copy of *He and I.* Opening it at the bookmark, I read these words of Christ: "Sing every day in your heart and make me known to others through joy." *Joy*—that was it! I had been focusing on my own unworthiness. After all, I reasoned, who was I to think our Lord was actually directing my involvement in this illness? Who was I, indeed, to expect God to perform a miracle for my friend? Asking for faith and discernment, I continued to read:

> Come to me. Show me your poor soul. Do as the sick folk in Judea did as I passed by: talk to me, beg me. The gospel says, "He healed them all." Quicken your faith and confidence. Speak to My extravagance of love and long to respond with your own.

A tingling sensation surged through my body. I knew that our tender, loving Lord was speaking to me once again through this book, the very book that He had chosen as one of many instruments to draw Phyllis and me closer. The significance of the statue had emanated from this jewel and I had no doubt that God was using it once again to let me know how very much He cared.

Phyllis was fascinated with the concept that God does indeed speak to us. I remember once saying to her, "Don't expect the phone to ring with a long distance operator announcing that God is calling you." Laughing, she responded, "Seriously, how *do* you know when it is God?"

"The only stumbling block is our unwillingness to listen," I insisted. "God speaks to us through others, through His Word in Holy Scripture—and through books like *He and I*." How prophetic those words turned out to be!

That same evening I called Jayne and shared my experience with her. Certainly the words "beg me" and "I healed them all" needed no interpretation. Was He turning my despair into joy? Maybe it was just me—was I indulging in wishful thinking? Was it as powerful as I thought?

"Absolutely," Jayne assured me. Then, unexpectedly, she confessed her own difficulty in praying for Phyllis. "Marion, in a state of frustration, I cried out and told God I simply could not pray. It was strange, almost as though He had been waiting for such an act of humble honesty, because I was immediately reminded of how your own mother walked away from cancer surgery!" Recalling

God's mercy in that instance, Jayne told me she was able to pray once again with confidence and expectant hope.

*   *   *

I don't use the word "miracle" lightly, but two extraordinary events had taken place in my own life that qualify as bona fide miracles. One, as I mentioned earlier, was the miraculous birth of my baby daughter which defied even the most sophisticated medical technology. The other came in the form of a pathology report on my mother declaring that there was no malignancy in her body—this, after she had already been through two biopsies, and had consulted three doctors whose findings all pointed to a lethal cancer, swift to spread.

I will never forget that Tuesday afternoon in Mercy Hospital as I sat beside Mother's bed waiting for the surgeon to make his rounds. She was slated to be operated on at 10:00 A.M. the following morning. Our concern was great because such radical surgery at her age, coupled with other medical problems, posed a serious risk. We avoided any discussion on the serious and disfiguring surgery she faced—it was easier to concentrate on harmless events from the past.

"He is so late today—I don't understand why," Mother said, somewhat nervously. Tired of sitting, I stood up and walked for a bit. The waiting, which had now stretched into three hours, was beginning to disturb me. Was something wrong?

No sooner had I returned to my chair when suddenly the doctor entered in the company of a young resident. Standing at the foot of Mother's bed, his tie askew, he cleared his throat. As he awkwardly ran his fingers through his hair, he shook his head in utter disbelief. "I'm late," he explained, "because the team of pathologists had a difficult time convincing me there was no cancer!"

Mother, who had been a nurse for thirty-five years,

stared at him as if he were a ghost. It was impossible for her to mentally shift gears that rapidly. She had expected the possibility of a spread to the colon and liver, and he said...what?

"Yes, Mrs. Lee, the pathologists unanimously agree that no cancer is present." Scratching his chin, he continued, "Myself, I have never known this type of lesion not to be malignant!"

Jolted from my former lethargy, I jumped out of the chair. "Doctor, do you believe in miracles?"

He smiled somewhat sheepishly.

"Well I do," I continued. "I've experienced one in my own life and I can recognize one when I see it."

His smile broadened and for an instant, whatever doubts he had seemed to disappear. However, following normal procedure, he said he would send to Boston for yet another opinion.

Just as he was leaving, the cleaning lady entered the room. Unable to conceal my joy, I blurted out the good news to her. This beautiful, uninhibited black woman, with mop in hand, began to praise out loud, "Sweet Jesus," and for a brief moment in time, we were all one with Him.

Mother was discharged immediately, and that evening, instead of keeping a vigil by her bedside, the family celebrated with a party. The laboratory results from Boston corroborated the findings in Pittsburgh. There was no sign of malignancy!

*   *   *

I am sure it was no accident that Jayne and I both had trouble praying for Phyllis. Because we turned to God with the problem, He helped us to help each other. Our part in Phyllis's journey was to support her in prayer. The prayers were vital and He wanted us to continue our efforts. The Lord's response to our requests was entirely His to give, in the manner in which He saw fit. Walking in that knowledge with the Lord is truly a "He and I" relationship.

When Phyllis picked up the results of the mammogram that afternoon, she called to tell me there was a shadow but no definite tumor according to the doctor.

After this turn of events, I confess I was somewhat apprehensive about having lunch with Phyllis. Having seen what I called the "cancer mask" in others with the disease, I fully expected a great physical change in her appearance. But to my great relief, she was still the stunning beauty she had always been—her physical appearance belied the destructive disease that was ravaging her internally.

Although we were more concerned with catching up on lots of news than with our food, I noticed that her appetite was good—fortunately, she was spared the awful sickness that often accompanies chemotherapy. "I do experience a slight nausea," she said, "but it never lasts long."

"How about pain?" I asked.

"No pain—discomfort and tenderness, but nothing I can't handle so far."

She had been living with this cancer for nearly two years, and the development and spread had been steady and unrelenting. The fact that she had suffered no pain and remained outwardly beautiful took on a symbolic significance for me. As long as she continued to look so well, I was able to delude myself into thinking she would never die.

Her plans were to continue with the treatment program and we kept in touch by telephone on a weekly basis. She did her best to stay calm despite the fact that there was no apparent improvement. By the end of March, a biopsy was performed on her remaining breast and the suspicious shadow was definitely a tumor. Another immediate concern was the inflammation on her chest which was not healing. She had no idea, when we spoke, what the next step would be—the news was too much for her to digest in a short time.

Her husband called a cancer hotline—he wanted another opinion. After carefully reviewing their options, they made the decision to go to Chicago where she was admitted into a hospital which specializes in the treatment and care of cancer patients. She went through a battery of tests and the results were not good: the inflammation was due to a staph infection. The tumor in the right breast was malignant, and there was another tumor in her shoulder, causing a great deal of swelling in her arm.

Phyllis began a regimen of five-day treatments, using a combination of conventional and experimental drugs. The potent chemicals she was now taking caused her to lose all her hair. There was a three-week interval between treatments, and she spent as much of that time as possible at home. As always, we kept in constant touch by phone. During one of our conversations, between her trips to Chicago, I noticed how labored her breathing sounded. It frightened me, and I found myself thinking, "She might be dying!"

"Oh no," I shuddered, "not Phyllis, she can't die!"

I later learned that the difficult breathing was a consequence of fluid building up in her lung. It was awful knowing she would have to go through the painful procedure of having that lung drained.

The Reminders

Bless the Lord, O my soul,
and forget not all His benefits.
Psalm 103:12

During Phyllis's third visit to Chicago, it was discovered that her white cell count was dangerously low. This made her chances for returning home in time for the college graduation of her son Mark, dismal. She couldn't bear the thought of lying in a hospital bed on this important day in his life. With only two days before the graduation, the situation appeared to be hopeless. Nevertheless, Elvira and I agreed to get together and pray the rosary.

We pleaded with God to grant this one request: make it possible for Phyllis somehow, some way, to get back to Pittsburgh in time. Elvira had been praying to Mary under her title of Queen of the Holy Angels. She suggested we ask Mary's intercession that God's angels accompany Phyllis and keep her safe from harm as she made her way through the now very difficult outside world. Words from Psalm 91 assured us that such a request was not only possible, but pleasing to the Lord:

> God will put his angels in charge of you
> to protect you wherever you go.
> Upon their hands they shall bear you up,
> lest you dash your foot against a stone.

The next day, Phyllis went home to Pittsburgh! She was too weak to attend the ceremony, but was able to share the rest of the day with Mark and her family. This small victory provided me with just enough encouragement not to give up but to continue to pray, and it confirmed in me the importance and power of intercessory prayer.

Phyllis was weak and tired but grateful to be home with her family, even though the care she had received at the hospital was excellent. One blessing was how well she continued to tolerate the chemicals—no vomiting or nausea. I counted that also as answered prayer. However, the swelling in her arm was getting worse and the pain intensifying.

Immediately upon her return to Chicago, the doctors started her on a new combination of chemotherapy. On June 25 she called to tell me that there was good news for a change. She was responding well—the swelling had actually left her hand and part of her forearm. Since the tumor was shrinking, the doctors wanted to continue with the drugs, but this meant she would have to stay longer in Chicago.

Phyllis never once called me without asking for prayers, and this was no exception. "Marion, I know all those wonderful people will pray. Please tell them to keep up the prayers...I need them." She had come to realize, as we came to see also, that every prayer was important, every answer lightened the burden, and, of course, with every request, there was a chance for a miracle.

A few days later, Phyllis called me again from Chicago. I no sooner finished saying hello when she began to cry. The swelling in her arm had returned. "Please pray for me, Marion. When you are lying here looking at the symptoms, it's easy to fall apart. I look at my body and I can't use either of my arms, my breast is shriveled up—I just need to sit and have a good cry. Thoughts come to my mind: 'Well, if praying is so great, why isn't it working?' I've been to so many healing services and it's getting worse. Then I keep remembering Larry and his faith."

"Phyllis, for heaven's sake, do you think he is superhuman?"

"He's more superhuman than I am," she cried.

"Nonsense," I said. "He would be just as frightened as you, and so would I!"

This was, by far, the most difficult conversation I ever had with Phyllis. Feeling totally inept, I inwardly begged God to give me the right words.

In mid-July, she went back home to Pittsburgh. Her sister Ann was there for a visit and answered the phone when I called. Within earshot of Phyllis, she didn't want to give me any new information. When I heard Phyllis's voice, she sounded extremely tired, but I could tell that her spirits were much better. In fact, I learned that she had encouraged Chuck to take the boys to California for a small vacation. This ordeal had robbed her family of a normal existence, and she was grateful for the opportunity to send them off with her blessing. Ann would stay on a few more days, and a close family friend had promised to come in until Chuck's return. Eventually, she planned to return to the hospital in Chicago.

"How long, Lord?" I thought. I was looking for a clue—any small sign—that might be a forerunner to a miracle. Then, the dear woman who had prayed with us at Larry's house popped into my mind. If anyone could encourage me, Nance could. After all, she had personally experienced what Phyllis was going through. At this point, I needed to be reminded of how she walked away from certain death. I got in touch with her and made no secret of my distress. Her voice was like balm, so soothing.

"There is no particular way the Lord heals. Why He chooses to heal some physically and not others, we do not know," she said. "There needs to be a healing of spirit and mind, too. I don't have any answers for you, Marion. God touched me the moment I said: 'I am broken, I am scared, I am tired'—words from my heart. And when I said, 'Either take me, or take me and use me,' I wasn't even sure what the word *use* meant. When I continued to live, I realized the

Lord had chosen to use me and no matter what happened, no matter what the doctors said, no matter how bad things looked—and they got worse before they got better—the Lord had other plans for me. If only Phyllis could look to the Lord and accept His plan for her. It might be a physical healing, a spiritual healing, or, perhaps, she will be an example to others. Believe in Him, Marion, He will take care of Phyllis in whatever He does or whatever happens to her."

In complete honesty, I confessed my fear that she might die. What disturbed me was, would it be possible under such circumstances to provide comfort and give her hope?

"I'm not hearing that!" Nance said. "Our purpose here is to prepare for everlasting life, and you *are* giving her the right words."

More than any time in the past, I was comforted to hear the details of Nance's story. As impressive as her physical healing was, the depth of her faith in God was a tonic for my tired mind. I prayed for more faith—the faith to believe a miracle was still possible, the faith to accept God's will in this matter.

The Valley

My God, my God, why have you
forsaken me?
Psalm 22:2

On Thursday, July 25, I learned that Phyllis had been
placed in Intensive Care. Almost immediately after Ann's
departure, she had taken a bad turn but somehow gathered
enough strength to board a plane for Chicago. Chuck
returned from California to be with her in the hospital; the
boys would drive the family car home to Pittsburgh and
join him the following weekend. It was her son Mark who
had called to give me the shocking news.

I remember sitting in my bedroom staring into space,
with the phone still cradled in my hand. What was it Nance
had said? "Believe in Him in whatever He does—in whatever happens...." That was easier said than done! Belief
to me was predicated on hope. Without hope, would I be
able to operate in faith? I was like a child playing hide and
seek with the Lord. I saw His hand in all the good news but
when things turned sour, it was as if He were non-
existent. Why wasn't God answering our prayers? I ques-
tioned all my prayers, all the prayers of the people here in
New Jersey, plus the people in Pittsburgh, and, of course,
the constant prayers of Phyllis's family. Were they doing
any good?

My husband was sitting at his desk in another room.
Having recently lost his own sister to the scourge of
cancer, Ed was familiar with the vicious assault this disease
can deal to its victims. As soon as he saw my face, he

realized something had gone wrong. "Phyllis?" he asked.

"Things look very bad," I said almost mechanically.

That night in bed, I tried to imagine Phyllis just where she was at that moment. A picture of a large hospital took shape—I saw long corridors and a gloss on the floor so bright it reflected one's image. The pungent odor of alcohol permeated the air. Two enormous doors swung open revealing the Intensive Care Unit, at the heart of which was the nurse's station. From this vantage point, each individual patient could be seen. Intensive Care Units, by their very nature, are not concerned with creating a cheerful ambiance; the scene I envisioned was no exception. It became so real to me, I could actually see a variety of life support systems, each with a different purpose, efficiently recording those bodily functions we normally take for granted. It was very quiet except for the continuous beep on the screens which were carefully monitored by the staff. Then I saw my beautiful friend, once the epitome of high fashion, lying helpless in a crude muslin gown.

"Oh Phyllis, you must be frightened by all that is happening to you! You can't even speak, dear friend, can you? Without that respirator, you can't even breathe!"

This morbid meandering became so vivid, I began to experience a heaviness in my chest. A sensation of oppression was closing in on me. Aware that I was merely conjuring up images while Phyllis was actually living this nightmare, I suddenly became moved to abject pity. My pillow was wet with tears as I begged God, "Please don't let her suffer!"

The vision still lingered in my mind when I awoke the next morning and I began projecting one fear onto another. My personal feelings colored all objectivity. With a heavy heart I called Elvira and Vada—I needed their strength at that moment. Each of them met this recent development with calm determination, holding fast to their belief that, even now, Phyllis could be healed.

Vada had been watching a Christian show on TV when I called, and she suggested I contact them and request prayers for Phyllis. "Maybe I'll do that," I said, but in my heart, I balked at the mere idea of calling an evangelical TV show for prayers. Somehow, it seemed undignified. After all, I reasoned, so many people were praying for Phyllis, and besides, that show was not Catholic. Then I thought, how ridiculous of me! Feeling properly ashamed, I reached for the phone.

A soft-spoken woman answered and I told her briefly what the situation was. I was moved to tears listening while this complete stranger uttered the most simple, sincere, yet profound prayer I had ever heard. The despair which had enveloped me like some dark impenetrable cloud evaporated and was replaced with a tranquility that covered me from head to toe like a warm caress from the sun. This lovely lady was more than a counselor—she managed to impart God's love and compassion to me. I sat quietly for the next few moments, not wanting to disturb the peace and joy that were now mine. Out of the corner of my eye, I noticed that my Bible, which had been left on the kitchen table, was open. I slid it over in front of me and my eyes fell upon Psalm 118, verses 19-24.

Open to me the gates of justice
I will enter them and give thanks
to the Lord.

This gate is the Lord's
the just shall enter it.

I will give thanks to you,
for you have answered me
and have been my Savior.

The stone which the builders rejected
has become the cornerstone.
By the Lord has this been done;
it is wonderful in our eyes.

This is the day the Lord has made;
let us be glad and rejoice in it.

The only phrase that stood out was "I will give thanks to you, for you have answered me and have been my Savior." Then I glanced at verses 15-18 of the same Psalm and read:

The joyful shout of victory
in the tents of the just.

The right hand of the Lord
has struck with power;
the right hand of the Lord is exalted;
the right hand of the Lord
has struck with power.

I shall not die, but live
and declare the works of the Lord.

Though the Lord has indeed chastised me,
yet He has not delivered me to death.

I couldn't believe what I had just read. I read it again, this time out loud. "Is this for Phyllis?" I cried. "Lord, I claim these words for Phyllis!" I had convinced myself that it was all over—and now this! The extraordinary words could not have been more explicit as far as I was concerned.

I grabbed the phone and called Vada. As soon as I heard her voice I exclaimed, "Oh Vada, the most incredible thing just happened!" I then told her how I had no intention of calling that TV show for prayer but, fortunately, a twinge of conscience prevailed over my self-righteousness.

"The woman I spoke with could not have been kinder or more empathetic—she also has a dear friend battling cancer—and her prayer lifted me right up from the pit!"

"That's beautiful!" Vada broke in.

"But wait, that's not all." And I excitedly told her about the Psalm, reading the passage to her and emphasizing the line, *"I shall not die, but live."*

"Isn't that amazing?" I squealed.

Vada responded with uncharacteristic excitement. "I

suggest you spend the rest of the day praising God!" she exclaimed.

"You can bet on that," I promised. "But first I must tell Elvira."

When I told Elvira, her reaction was exactly the same as mine. Both of us reveled in this eleventh-hour word from the Lord. He was going to deliver Phyllis! Despite the grim circumstances, He who has authority over every situation would strike with power! My struggle would be to patiently wait for His intervention.

There is a very thin line between trust and presumption, and I wanted so much to believe that Phyllis would be healed. Knowing how wishful thinking can make one create God in one's own fantasy, I asked for a sign—a confirmation—that the words were indeed from Him and that they were directly concerned with raising Phyllis from her deathbed.

The Butterfly

I am the Resurrection and the Life.
He who believes in me...will never die.
John 11:26

The paradox of the passage, *"I shall not die but live,"* was puzzling to be sure. But I was confident that soon those words would be confirmed, and then the mystery of suffering would pale in comparison to the miracle of her healing. But by the end of the week there was no change, and my resolve was beginning to crumble.

At Mass on Sunday, I listened intently to every word of the readings, secretly anticipating that Psalm 118 might be repeated. Then I realized how foolish my behavior was—I had asked God for a sign but I was trying to choose how and what that sign would be. I had to remind myself that God's ways are not our ways.

When Mass was over, I stayed and offered a rosary for Phyllis. Meditating on the Divine Mysteries, I asked to be preserved from the sin of presumption, to be blessed with enough grace to accept God's will. Emotionally tossed about in a sea of confusion, I prayed, "Lord, you know how desperately I want her to live. Please help me to understand what is happening."

My solitude was interrupted by the sound of happy voices in the front of the church. While I was pleading with God to spare the life of one of His precious creations, new life was being celebrated in the sacrament of Baptism. In the midst of such joy, my tears seemed out of place, so I quietly slipped out of church.

Walking to my car in the now almost empty parking lot, a beautiful butterfly, white and pale yellow and outlined with black, swooped down in front of my face. It gracefully landed on the hood of my car, rested there for a few moments, then flew away.

"How beautiful!" I said aloud. The words were hardly out of my mouth when it struck me. "Could *this* be your sign, Lord?" In an instant, I was reminded of how butterflies had once before played a part in my life.

*   *   *

It had happened just prior to the death of my only nephew, David, who was born with cystic fibrosis. When he was thirteen, he spent his last Thanksgiving holiday with my family. Saying goodbye, somehow I knew I would never see him again. The last thing he spoke of was a surprise he was making for Katie. "It's almost finished!" he told me proudly. I was touched to realize that he was spending his final days thinking of another child.

Shortly after that day, a rumpled package, wrapped in brown paper, arrived in the mail. Inside was a beautiful, brightly-colored mobile of butterflies made with construction paper. This gift is one of Katie's prized possessions and hangs from the ceiling in her bedroom.

Our dear David died that following Easter Sunday—the day of the Resurrection.

*   *   *

Standing there in the parking lot, I was again reminded that the butterfly was considered a sign of the resurrection, but I disregarded that thought immediately. I didn't want to think about Phyllis's "resurrection"—I wanted her to live!

August first—my baby Katie's birthday once again, and the anniversary of Phyllis's visit. It was important to me that this anniversary be marked with special prayers of thanksgiving and intercession. Therefore, I invited the same women to come to my home who had shared in such a special way with Phyllis the year before.

The birthday festivities kept the children occupied and this allowed the mothers to join hands in prayer. We thanked God for the past year and lifted up Phyllis to Him in this, her hour of greatest need. The significance of the date served to intensify the small hope still burning inside of me. One year ago Phyllis had been prayed for by Larry, renewed in the Holy Spirit, and told it was her time to receive gifts. I felt in my heart that the time was perfect for God to touch her once again—to heal Phyllis this very day.

However, I had no word from Pittsburgh or Chicago that day, but "No news is good news," I thought.

On August 5, another old and cherished friend, Rose, called me long distance. She told me that, in July, while visiting her mother in Pittsburgh, she had gone to see Phyllis—just a few days before Phyllis's sudden turn for the worse. Rose told me how reluctant she had been to make this visit, afraid of what she might find. To her astonishment, Phyllis looked radiant and was thrilled she had come.

"Marion, she put me totally at ease with her delightful wit and humor." Then, with a painful sigh, Rose added, "I can't believe she was placed in intensive care just two days after I saw her."

"Outwardly, she was still so beautiful," Rose continued. "The only indication of how ill she is came when I touched her hand and kissed her cheek. Her body was icy cold and it frightened me."

Unsettled about the ultimate outcome myself, I wasn't able to tell her the "good news" I had received from the psalm. Instead, I recounted the story of the statue. Repeating the statue story to anyone who was unaware of it always strengthened my own faith, and this proof of God's loving concern bolstered Rose's spirits immediately.

"How's that for ingenuity?" I asked. "Imagine God doing such a marvelous thing for Phyllis! We have to trust and believe He is watching over her."

After talking to Rose, I had an urgent desire to call the hospital in Chicago. Naturally, Phyllis would be unable to talk but she could still receive messages. On second thought, I decided it might be better to call her sister Ann first.

The tone of Ann's voice made it obvious that she had resigned herself to the loss of her baby sister. The thought came to me that if Ann, a beautiful woman with a deep and abiding faith, felt Phyllis would die, who was I to indulge my imagination with fantasies of a miraculous, last-minute cure? What gave me the right to think God would bless me with subtle hints of something so contrary to the reality of the situation?

It wasn't that I couldn't accept her death. For me, it was a crisis of faith; I wanted to know what was happening on a spiritual level. The words I had received, all the touches and experiences of those of us who had prayed with and for Phyllis—all of this seemed to indicate a miraculous healing. Yet she continued to grow weaker.

The next evening Ann called me with more bad news. Phyllis was fading rapidly. It could be a matter of hours now—the doctors felt she would not last the week. No pain, thank God, and she was still conscious, but Ann wanted to prepare me for the final phone call. I was deeply moved by her charity because I knew how tragic this was for her personally.

As devastating as this news was, Elvira and I decided to pray the rosary together. We offered it in thanksgiving for the way our own lives had been affected and for all that God had done and would continue to do for Phyllis.

August 8—another milestone. Not only was it my birthday, but it was the twenty-sixth wedding anniversary of Phyllis and Chuck. I tried not to give in to the fear and anxiety that Phyllis might die on this day. In order to keep myself occupied, I spent the day shopping with my mother at a nearby mall. In one of the shops, I ran into an elderly couple who occasionally came to our prayer meetings. We chatted for a while, then I told them how deeply concerned I was because my beloved friend was dying. It was extremely difficult for me to utter these words. Alluding to her imminent death seemed to be almost a betrayal. They promised to remember her in their prayers and I knew it would be a promise fulfilled.

Just before leaving the mall, Mother and I decided to browse in our favorite gift shop. Spotting a table filled with different gift items marked "clearance," I eagerly walked over to see what was on sale. As I approached the table, I stopped abruptly. There, right in front of me, was a beautiful white and pale yellow butterfly outlined in black— exactly like the one I had seen that day in the parking lot! This one was mounted in a gold frame, and I knew I had to have it for myself. Maybe it had some special purpose, maybe not, but even though my senses were somewhat fraught with worry, I still had a vague feeling that God was trying to tell me something through this butterfly. The minute we got home, I hung it on the wall in the entrance hall. I wanted it to be the first thing anyone would see as they entered the front door.

The following day I had lunch with one of the women who had been at my home on Katie's birthday. She told me that when we had prayed that day, it was the first and only time she had felt an anointing while praying for Phyllis. (An anointing is an involuntary sensation, sometimes a feeling of warmth, and usually reveals the power of the Holy Spirit at work.) This was startling news because another friend who had been there that day told me the same thing. Was their experience a confirmation of my own perception? Was He preparing their hearts for a miracle?

I knew that now was the time to call the hospital. The switchboard put me through to ICU where a friendly, courteous nurse answered the phone. Regretfully, she was unable to give me any information, but she assured me that Phyllis was conscious and she would happily give her a message from me. "Please tell her that Marion called to say I love you very much and I am praying for you constantly."

Later that evening, the elderly woman I had met at the mall and who had promised to pray for Phyllis, called to inquire if she had "expired." She said, "I've prayed all day for her—a very simple prayer. I asked Jesus to reveal Himself to your friend, to be with her in that hospital room. I haven't been able to get her out of my mind."

Her concern and the fact that she had taken the time to call me meant so very much. The motivating power that compelled so many people to pray for Phyllis—and not only to pray, but to be genuinely interested in her—was still in operation.

The Gathering

A time to weep, a time to laugh;
a time to mourn and a time to dance.
Ecclesiastes 3:4

In the early morning of August 12, 1985, God took
Phyllis from us. Chuck, Mark and Kevin, were at her
bedside until she slipped into a final coma.

When the news reached me, I was bewildered more than
shocked. After all, Ann had prepared me, and all signs
indicated this would happen. But it was the other signs, the
signs of the past two years that I didn't understand. What
meaning did they have? Why did God go to so much trouble and why were so many people involved, if not to bring
about a miracle? It just didn't seem to make sense.

Because her body had to be transported from Chicago to
Pittsburgh, the funeral was delayed. Ann called when the
final arrangements were in order. Ed and I made plans to
stay with old friends, Nancy and Bob, who would also be
going to the funeral.

Preparations before funerals are a blessing in disguise—
they keep one's mind busy. A Mass card had to be prepared
and flowers had to be sent ahead. I wanted personally to
select an arrangement—nothing elaborate, but something
that would in some way reflect Phyllis. We had no success
in the first florist shop. None of the standard arrangements struck my fancy. On our next stop, I was poring
over the pages in the catalog when the owner, seeing my
dismay, asked if she could help in any way.

"I'm looking for something special for a dear and precious friend," I explained. "I'll know it when I see it, but I can't seem to find just what I want."

She hesitated a moment, then went to the back and brought out another book, an old catalog. After glancing through a few pages, I found the perfect arrangement, but now the problem was whether or not it was still available. The owner was genuinely compassionate—she sensed how important this was to me. After making a long-distance phone call, she promised me it could be made to order. So I chose yellow roses and white mums with a delicate white statue of the Blessed Mother nestled in the middle. It was the Madonna that had caught my eye—we had relied on Mary's intercession so many times during the illness, and Phyllis had such devotion to her.

Coincidentally, the following day was the Feast of the Assumption of our Blessed Mother. Ed and I attended an early Mass and then set out for Pittsburgh. During the drive, I found it hard to believe Phyllis was gone—it just wasn't sinking in, and I desperately wanted my feelings to catch up with reality. I suppose this is a common experience in grief—a sort of blissful cushion against unbearable pain.

We arrived at Nancy and Bob's late in the afternoon. This was going to be a difficult time for all of us, and it was comforting to be able to share our sorrow. We had just enough time to shower and eat before going to the funeral home. Nancy, normally so vivacious and gregarious, was very subdued. While I was putting on my makeup, she stood by the doorway in the hall. "The casket is going to be closed," she said.

When I asked how she knew that, Nancy replied that one of Phyllis's sisters had told her—but she didn't know anymore than that.

"Phyllis must have looked pretty bad at the end, if that's the case," I said. Selfishly, I longed to see her beautiful face, just one more time. Maybe Nancy was wrong, I told myself.

We drove to the funeral home in Bob's car, nervously filling the time with superficial chatter. By the time we reached our destination, I could feel the anxiety in every part of my being. The entrance hall was packed with people and I busily scanned the crowd looking for a familiar face.

My old friend Sally, the one who had taken Phyllis to the prayer meetings at St. Thomas More Church, and her husband Jim spotted us and came right over. Words were unnecessary with Sally—like me, she had become deeply involved in Phyllis's illness. We talked briefly, then Ed and I made our way into the waiting room. Phyllis's sister Ann came over to us and I kissed her cheek and told her how very sorry I was. Our common love for Phyllis had brought us together during her illness and had left an indelible mark on each of us. There was nothing we could, or had to say to each other.

Looking around, I noticed that there were flowers everywhere—in the reception area, the waiting room, and surrounding the room that held the casket. Some of the arrangements were magnificent, but I felt especially honored because our humble offering was set up on a small pedestal table all alone.

Ed took my hand and together we walked into the room where the casket was. Chuck was standing a few feet away from the casket. The minute he saw us, he came forward and, with tears in his eyes, embraced me. "I loved her so much," he said, weeping.

It took all the strength I had to keep my composure as he escorted us both to the coffin where we knelt down together to pray. It *was* closed, with not even a picture nearby. "This can't be real," I thought. "If only I could look at her once more, I might be able to say what's in my heart. And yet, if I saw her face, perhaps it would be unbearable."

But Chuck explained to us later that the closed casket

had nothing to do with Phyllis's appearance. "Her beautiful face was never marred," he said. The reason it was closed was to honor a lifelong promise he had made to her: she wanted people always to remember her alive.

Ed tenderly took my arm and we made our way back to the waiting room. I spied my friend Rose in the crowd—the one who had called me to tell me about her visit to Phyllis a few days before her admission to the Intensive Care Unit. As soon as our eyes met, Rose shook her head in disbelief— for the past thirty years, our reunions had always been happy ones. Now, she had traveled from her home in Virginia, and I from New Jersey, to be reunited by the death of our beloved Phyllis.

Rose and I did our best to console each other, but the hurt was so deep. With tear-stained cheeks, she smiled gently and said, "Everyone teases me about the dreams I have, but I had a dream last night that was so eerie! You remember, Marion, I told you how icy cold Phyllis was when I saw her?"

"Yes, I remember," I whispered.

"Well, in my dream, a man entered my room and Phyllis was with him. She came over to my bed smiling. She bent down, kissed me on the forehead, and said, 'See, Rose, I told you I would be all right.' Marion, what I noticed most was her body—it exuded warmth!"

"Who was the man?" I asked. Without a word, her eyes conveyed the unmistakable message: "Who do you think?"

Because there were so many people paying their respects, Chuck didn't have very much time to spend with us. He asked Ed and me to come to his home later that evening. He was obviously tired, but, realizing his need for our comforting support, we told him we would come over for a short visit.

Entering the house through the back porch, we stepped into the breakfast nook. I had forgotten how elegant this room was. I used to tease Phyllis that her home always looked ready for a magazine layout. Still picture perfect, it was hauntingly empty without her. Every direction I looked in reminded me of her.

I noticed Phyllis's brother and sister, Jim and Rita, talking in the dining room. Their grief had to be magnified by the fact that Phyllis was the baby in the family—it's an unnatural turn of events to bury a baby sister. We found Chuck in the living room chatting with a few friends. He came over immediately, invited us to sit down, and pulled up a chair beside us. He looked weary, but there was a need to talk about the last days.

"Marion," he said, "I would never have gone to California if I thought Phyllis was going to take such a bad turn. She insisted I take the boys for a few days."

"I know Chuck, I know. She was happy because you and the boys were able to get away for awhile."

He continued, "You knew that August 8 was our wedding anniversary—I wanted somehow to make the day a little festive, so after an early breakfast with the boys, I stopped at a flower shop. We arrived at the hospital with a card and a single rose. She was on the respirator, unable to speak, so I wrote a note telling her how much we loved her. She looked at the three of us, nodded and smiled. There was such a peace about her—all that fear was gone!"

It was then that he told me how her body was consumed with cancer. There were even visible tumors on her back and shoulders, and yet her face never changed in color or appearance. Chuck had done everything he possibly could to save Phyllis, but toward the end he let go, accepting God's will—not in anger but humility.

It was hard to sleep that night. Nancy and I stayed up, going over and over every detail. It was the first opportunity we had to talk privately. She had no idea of my present spiritual struggle when she remarked, "It was good Phyllis could talk to you throughout this ordeal."

"Yes," I agreed somewhat reluctantly, "but it was also a

great burden. There were times when I felt completely inadequate to the task."

"She was such a private person. Maybe it was because you lived in another city that she turned to you."

"That may have been the reason in the beginning," I admitted. "But as things progressed, she came to rely on me and I was so afraid of letting her down."

I then told Nancy how, during one of Phyllis's visits, she had even joked about the reliance she had on me. Phyllis had a wonderful sense of humor—it wasn't what she said, it was her delivery that turned a casual remark into something hilarious. My husband Ed had asked her a simple question, but shaking her head in mock dismay, she motioned towards me as she told him, "You'll have to check with my spiritual advisor!"

Nancy smiled in recognition. She knew how droll Phyllis could be, and, when the occasion warranted, what a genius she had for facial expressions.

It was impossible to relate to Nancy everything that had happened from my perspective. Nevertheless, I shared with her the words from Psalm 118—the words I had thought meant that Phyllis was to live. "Nancy, at the time I actually thought these words were from the Holy Spirit. I used to fantasize her rising from that hospital bed, healed and whole. I could even see the reaction on the faces of all who knew her!"

Undaunted, Nancy replied, "I'm sure the Holy Spirit directed you to that psalm, however, I think you misinterpreted the meaning. Those words tell me about the resurrection of Phyllis."

There was that word again, resurrection! Still, the full impact of what she was saying did not hit me, but God was planting a seed in my mind that night.

Scripture says that we see through a glass darkly. Throughout the funeral Mass, I tried in vain to find some hidden meaning, some purpose to God's plan. But as we knelt together in sorrow, I was able to find reason to rejoice: so many childhood friends had been brought together in this time of sorrow. For as long as I can remember, people have marveled at the fact that all these friends had managed to remain so close. This bond, I am convinced, was a special gift from God, a reflection of His love. That thought has always been and continues to be a joy in times of gladness and a comfort in times of grief.

During the Mass, when the priest uttered the words, "...on earth as it is in heaven," I realized that although he was unable to paint a portrait of the Phyllis we knew, he was correct about the importance of praying for her soul. We, her friends on earth, would continue to pray for the soul of Phyllis. And I honestly believed she would intercede for us with all the saints in heaven. Inspired by this beautiful thought, I asked Phyllis that day, and many times since then, to thank God personally for allowing me to be part of such a beautiful bond.

*   *   *

Grief cannot be denied for long—there must be a release. After the funeral, Ed and I returned home, packed the kids in the car and left for a week's vacation. Even though I was occupied with lots of sightseeing, my mind was still on the cutting edge of sadness. I kept crying out to God, "Why? Why did you allow me to become so involved? What good did it do?" I had given lip service often enough in the past to Him about trusting in His plan. That was easy to do when Phyllis was alive and I had entertained fantasies that she would be a living witness to the power of God. Now that she was gone, I wondered, what was the purpose of my role?

There were friends back in New Jersey who would want to hear about the funeral. But when we returned from vacation, I was so low I didn't want to see or talk to anyone.

The following Sunday after Mass, Elvira saw me and came over to my car. There was now no way to avoid a conversation. When she asked me about the funeral, I moaned, "It's just beginning to sink in and I'm very depressed." She gently took my hand and squeezed it. "I understand," she said. "Come over tomorrow—we'll talk."

I practically had to drag myself to her house the next day. We sat at the kitchen table—the same spot where we had prayed for Phyllis so many times. I spread several prayer cards from the funeral on the table, and asked Elvira to choose one. On a positive note, I told her how much Chuck had emphasized the fact that Phyllis had no fear. But in describing the funeral itself, I broke down—I couldn't speak.

Elvira got up from her chair and came over to put her arms around me. Praying out loud, she pleaded with God to reveal the why and wherefore of it all to me.

Later that week, I had lunch with Jayne. She was anxious to hear every detail leading up to and including the funeral. She knew how hopeful I had been that Phyllis would survive, and how it was that hope that had kept me going.

"Why did God continue to encourage me?" I sighed.

Jayne has what I call "Holy Boldness." With a rock solid faith, and the faculty of getting right to the heart of the matter, she looked at me intensely as she said, "Marion, God chose you because He trusted you with Phyllis."

What a beautiful thing to say! The lump in my throat began to ache and I could no longer fight the tears. "If only I could believe that..."

"Believe it!" Jayne repeated firmly.

These dear friends who had comforted Phyllis with prayers were now comforting me. There were others I needed to see—most especially Larry and Vada. I told them that Chuck had singled out Larry twice while I was in Pittsburgh. In fact, his parting words were, "Marion, please thank that man Larry. He meant so much to Phyllis.

He was such a comfort to her." Obviously touched, Larry smiled.

I asked him, "Didn't you, like me, think Phyllis was going to be healed? Her condition certainly went from bad to worse, but the day I got those words from Psalm 118—'I shall not die, but live'—it seemed so obvious."

With an expression of sadness, Larry spoke, "Yes I did. But in our human desire, we can and do make false assumptions—it's happened to me. God's will and way has a purpose. Ask Him to reveal it to you."

"That is exactly how Elvira prayed for me." I replied. "Right now, the pain is too near—perhaps some day I'll understand more clearly."

Larry was no stranger to accepting God's will. His experience in the healing ministry had taught him humility in the face of God's power. He now took my hand and reached over to Vada, inviting her to join hands with us. He prayed for Phyllis first, then for each of us, praising God for all that He had done. It was a very moving moment.

Suddenly, I realized that if it hadn't been for Phyllis, I might never have come to know these wonderful people who had become very dear to me. It was important to me that Larry, Vada, and all the kind people who had prayed for Phyllis knew how appreciative I was. After all, my concern was natural; their's was something special—and that "something special" had to be the continuous outpouring of God's grace. To the very end, they had prayed unceasingly. I have to admit that had I known the outcome, I would never have been able to pray with enthusiasm.

I came to see that, through Phyllis, God was able to touch many lives and to enliven the faith of all those whose lives were touched. And she will continue to live through us here as a result of God's kindness. We—all of us—are on a journey to eternity. Yes, I mourn the loss of a precious friend, but my suffering is overpowered by the certain knowledge of life eternal.

The Answer

The recesses of the darkness He discloses,
and brings the gloom forth to the light.
Job 12:22

Several years ago, my husband and I spent a weekend with Chuck and Phyllis at their home. I remember something Phyllis said on that occasion that has more meaning now than it had at the time. We were enjoying our usual "girl talk" gab session when I shared with her an experience that seemed to be more than coincidental. She listened attentively, then told me emphatically, "There are no accidents—it's all part of a plan!"

You're right, dear friend, there are no accidents.

At this moment, I'm gazing out through my back porch door, and my eyes can see only those trees which are directly within my range of vision. We catch only small glimpses of God's glory in nature because our vision is limited. The same holds true with God's supernatural touches. However, the more we try to come closer to the Lord, the more He reveals Himself to us.

Eye has not seen, ear has not heard
nor has it so much as dawned on man
what God has prepared for those
who love Him.
Yet God has revealed this wisdom
to us through the Spirit!

The first day I heard the awful news that Phyllis had cancer, it did not dawn on me how much God was willing to reveal Himself. In the beginning of her illness I was uncertain, doubtful, even at times fearful, but with each message from God, no matter what form it took, my faith grew. Now I can look back and realize there were no accidents.

God loves each of us so intensely, so perfectly. I stand in awe of His powerful majesty. He knew I had to get past my sorrow before I could savor His goodness. With the passage of time, ever so slowly and gently, He helped me to recall all the loving kindnesses He had shown me.

Phyllis was the instrument God used to teach so many the importance of intercessory prayer. When she first became ill, I pleaded for a miracle. But sometimes we concentrate so much on a physical healing, we lose sight of what God is doing. To begin with, He allowed me the privilege of comforting my dear friend in her time of need. Never relying on my own resources, I called out to God and He answered me, giving me the words to console her.

The first hint of God's plan for Phyllis began, I believe, with my visit to the Shrine of St. Anne de Beaupré. There, the power of the Holy Spirit gently taught me that intercessory prayer does not die and that the Communion of Saints is alive and well. Years before, Phyllis had recommended St. Anne to me as intercessor; through the grace of the Holy Spirit, I was reminded at the Shrine that my request had been heard and answered. This was the motivating factor that created in me such a compelling desire to pray conscientiously.

At Madison Square Garden, we saw Christ's healing power manifested in a dramatic way. I believe Phyllis was healed in some way that day, perhaps known only to God. His Word does not return to Him void.

When she came to New Jersey, I had a real taste of God's perfect goodness. I asked our Lord to take charge of the visit, and He did, beginning with the women who each shared their own unique story of how God had met them in their need. Everyone involved played a crucial role, every sentence had a purpose, every detail built onto the next.

The night we went to Larry's home, Phyllis experienced Christ's love and concern through the humble obedience of a few faithful servants who were not afraid to put the Gospel into action. Then, at the prayer meeting, the inspired request by Kathy that a new infilling of the Holy Spirit be granted to Phyllis was a reassurance that God's Holy Spirit was present and overshadowing her.

Her sister Ann was inspired too, I am sure, when she arranged the delightful surprise visit to the Shrine of St. John Neumann. The experience was so good for Phyllis— the thought of his intercession on her behalf was a source of great hope to her.

The discovery of our common appreciation of *He and I* proved to be more than a coincidence. It was that very book that God used to reach out and touch her emotionally when she saw the holy card of the "Palm of His Hand" inside.

And who but our wonderful God could have steered her to a Healing Mass in a neighboring parish, setting the stage to present her with the gift that Larry had prophesied she would receive—the gift being that very "Palm of His Hand" statue.

That statue was a blessing to her, and to those of us who were praying for her, it was a constant source of encouragement. Prayer was our means of reaching up to God. By providing the statue, He reached down to all of us.

The power of prayer cannot be measured. As we here on earth pray for the living and the dead, those who have died pray for us. Even Jesus Himself pleads on our behalf to the Father:

> ...Christ Jesus, who died, or rather
> who was raised to life and is at the
> right side of God, pleading with him for us! (*Romans 8:34*)

And so he is able, now and always,
to save those who come to God through Him,
because He lives forever to plead with
God for them.   (*Hebrews 7:25*)

...We have someone who pleads with the
Father on our behalf—Jesus Christ,
the righteous one.   (*1 John 2:1*)

He listened to all of our prayers, and each and every
prayer was important. He healed Phyllis—not of cancer,
but of all fear, all anxiety, and with His gentle hand He
carried her home. This was His plan from the beginning,
although my eyes were blinded to the truth.

And when in my blindness, I made my urgent cry to God,
I am certain His response through Psalm 118 was no
accident.

The joyful shout of victory
in the tents of the just.

The right hand of the Lord
has struck with power:
The right hand of the Lord is exalted;
The right hand of the Lord
has struck with power.

I shall not die, but live,
and declare the works of the Lord.

Though the Lord has indeed chastised me
Yet He has not delivered me to death.

Open to me the gates of justice;
I will enter then and give
thanks to the Lord.

This gate is the Lord's;
The just shall enter it.

I will give thanks to you,

for you have answered me and
have been my Savior.

The stone which the builders rejected
has become the cornerstone.
By the Lord has this been done;
It is wonderful in our eyes.

This is the day the Lord has made;
Let us be glad and rejoice in it.

(*Psalm 118:15-24*)

God was telling me that Phyllis would enter His gates. And three times His hand is mentioned in that passage. Why didn't I recognize it when I first read those words? In my human weakness and desire to have God do things my way, I just wasn't listening.

But God, in His tenderness, tried to communicate with me again through the gift of the butterfly perched on my car. He had used the symbol of the butterfly once before, in the case of my nephew David, and knew I would understand its significance. But when I saw the butterfly that Sunday morning after praying for Phyllis, I chose to dismiss its real meaning—as a sign of the Resurrection. I simply wasn't willing to accept His plan.

And then how patient God was with me—gently leading me to that gift shop where I saw the exact replica of the butterfly. Knowing I had misinterpreted the words in the psalm, He lovingly tried to put me back on the right path.

After the funeral, it was Elvira first, then Larry, who prayed so earnestly, asking the Lord to reveal His purpose to me. And once again, God in His infinite love made His presence known in our lives by answering their prayers in an extraordinary way.

Several months following Phyllis's death, God opened my eyes to what was always within my grasp—in my grief, it had escaped me. The day she had received the statue, I knew God had done something wonderful, not only for

Phyllis, but for me and for all who shared in the prayers. What I couldn't possibly know then was the significance of the day itself on which God had chosen to reveal Himself to her in such a personal way.

You see, on August 12, 1984, God arranged for Phyllis to receive the statue—His proof that she was cradled in the palm of His hand.

On August 12, 1985, with great tenderness and love, God cradled Phyllis in the palm of His hand and took her home.

ALLELUIA!

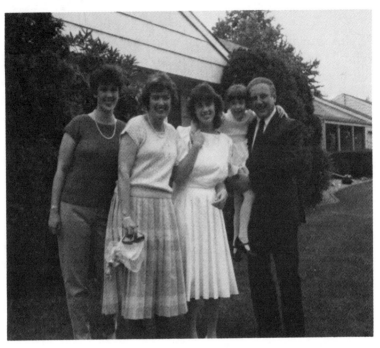

Left to right: Ellen, Marion, Liz, Katie and Ed

The author was born Marion Lee in Pittsburgh, PA in 1936. She married Edward Levandowski in 1963 and they have three daughters: Ellen, Liz, and Katie. It was the birth of Katie that brought Marion national attention with her story, "A Miracle Called Katie," which was published in *Good Housekeeping* magazine in June of 1982.

A full-time homemaker, she has also been a CCD teacher, a telephone counselor, and an officer on the board of Burlington County Right to Life.

In addition to her writing, Marion has appeared on television promoting the pro-life message and has been a guest speaker for various organizations.

OTHER TITLES FROM ST. BEDE'S

Spirituality Recharted   *Hubert van Zeller*
In this delightful book, Dom Hubert presents one of his favorite
themes: "the pursuit of sanctity by responding to the grace of
spirituality." The method of approach is basically that of putting
into everyday language St. John of the Cross's treatment of the
soul's progress toward union with God. A best-seller!
Paperback, 157 pages   **$4.95**

By Death Parted   *Philip Jebb, editor*
Six widows from England share with you the accounts of their
first years of widowhood and how they learned to cope with the
loneliness and problems of being "suddenly single." The book
offers consolation as well as practical advice for all who have
been recently widowed. A wonderful gift for a friend.
Paperback, 101 pages   **$5.95**

Widowed   *Philip Jebb*
A sourcebook for the widowed. The author touches on practical
problems while developing a spirituality of widowhood, pointing
out that the Church itself has been a widow since the ascension
of Christ. A grandson of Hilaire Belloc, Father Jebb has inherited
his grandfather's trenchant and fascinating style. Makes a
wonderful gift.
Paperback, 90 pages   **$3.95**

Victory Over Death   *Ronda Chervin*
This beautiful book is meant for all of us, to show us that nothing
in the world can compare with the joys of heaven. It will help you
to deal with all aspects of death—your own or that of a loved
one—and offers suggestions for developing your own prepara-
tion for *Victory Over Death.*
Paperback, 63 pages   **$3.95**

Reflections   *Charles Rich*
A book of profound yet simple spiritual wisdom for all interested
in personal growth in holiness. The author, a lay contemplative,
leads you through various aspects of the spiritual life such as the
meaning of suffering, the nature of prayer, and being one with
Christ. This book will help you to focus on the ultimate
reality—God.
Paperback, 131 pages   **$6.95**

Gateway to Hope: An Exploration of Failure

Maria Boulding, OSB

Learning to deal with failure is a part of life, says the author. Drawing on the Bible and on human experience, she shows that in our failure lies our success. Weakness, sin, death itself have all been overcome, for in the ultimate failure—the Cross—we see the greatest triumph of both man and God: the gateway to our hope and to the glory that awaits us.

Paperback, 158 pages   **$5.95**

The Wheel of Becoming: Personal Growth through the Liturgical Year

Augustin Belisle, OSB

Reflecting on the seasonal cycle of the liturgical year, the author presents insights into the rhythms and seasons of everyone's journey through the mysteries of Christ, and helps you to understand more clearly how these mysteries are directly connected with your growth as a human person.

Paperback, 87 pages   **$6.95**

Hammer and Fire: The Way to Contemplative Happiness, Fruitful Ministry, and Mental Health in Accordance with the Judeo-Christian Tradition

Raphael Simon, OCSO, MD

Many people today are seeking guidance, but are confused by the various methods of spirituality being presented to them. *Hammer & Fire* instructs us in the Gospel path of transformation in Christ through prayer and meditation, in accordance with sound doctrine, Scripture, Tradition, and the principles of mental health and personal development. The book not only attempts to set up a program of spiritual direction for the lay person, but also provides principles of direction for priests, religious, and all who are called upon to counsel others. It is a profound and very complete guide.

Paperback, 268 pages   **$9.95**

Order From:

St. Bede's Publications
P.O. Box 545
Petersham, MA 01366-0545

Prices subject to change without notice
Send for our complete catalog of books and tapes.